STEVE MILLER'S
SLIMMING SECRETS

STEVE MILLER'S SLIMMING SECRETS

metro

Published by Metro Publishing
an imprint of John Blake Publishing Ltd
3 Bramber Court, 2 Bramber Road,
London W14 9PB, England

www.johnblakepublishing.co.uk

www.facebook.com/Johnblakepub facebook
twitter.com/johnblakepub twitter

First published in paperback in 2012

ISBN: 978-1-84358-789-7

British Library Cataloguing-in-Publication Data:

A catalogue record for this book is available from the British Library.

Design by www.envydesign.co.uk

Printed in Great Britain by CPI Group (UK) Ltd, Croydon, CR0 4YY

1 3 5 7 9 10 8 6 4 2

Papers used by John Blake Publishing are natural,
recyclable products made from wood grown in sustainable forests.
The manufacturing processes conform to the environmental
regulations of the country of origin.

Every attempt has been made to contact the relevant copyright-
holders, but some were unobtainable. We would be grateful if
the appropriate people could contact us.

I dedicate this book to the memory of my special friend June Linda Thompson, who inspired me to believe it was all possible.

CONTENTS

ACKNOWLEDGEMENTS

I would like to thank the following people for making this book possible: Alan Possart for his constant support and for putting up with me in more ways than one. Terry Brookes for his support and friendship, and for making the best cup of tea in the world. Alison Carman, a fantastic consultant nutritionist, for her support in making things real world. My beloved cats, Jack and Jamie, who sadly passed away recently – I still hear you purr! My mum and dad, who raised me in such a way to help make my dreams come true. My Auntie Margaret, who sadly passed away – she supported me from a young boy. Amy and Ryan, my niece and nephew, who are the apples of my eyes. Blax and Minnie, my cats, who still run around while I'm writing. Lindsey Gibson, my stylist, who helps to keep me looking crisp. Jean Wilde for being such a great mate and believing in me. Matt Rowland for, once again, playing his part so well. Thanks to Sara Cywinski, my editor. The Bell Lomax Moreton Agency for helping to make it happen. Kirsty Milner and Vicki Mellor at Billy Marsh. All my wonderful friends and clients and finally to you, enjoy the book!

'What's wonderful about the future is that we can change; something you can never do in the past.'

Steve Miller

HOW I FOUND MY OWN SECRETS

It's 1999 and I'm driving down the motorway when suddenly my heart begins to pound. I become dizzy and have to pull over onto the hard shoulder. Life has become all too much as blood and emotions course through my body. There's a whirlwind tying my stomach in knots and my head feels like a time bomb about to explode. That was the day of reckoning for me, over fifteen years ago, and it was to mark the beginning of my own radical life change. I resigned from a well-paid job, took action to sort out my flagging confidence and took a long, hard look in the mirror. And then, in no uncertain terms, I told myself to do something about the gut-busting barrel I'd become.

I'd 'tried' many times to lose weight before, but all previous attempts to shed the flab had come to nothing as I carried on eating too much, enjoyed far too many take-aways and couldn't be bothered to get my backside off the sofa and do some exercise. Like many people, I'd munched my way through tons of salad and followed loads of faddy diets only to fail after the first few weeks. I even went down the route of getting a 'helping hand' by joining slimming clubs, but they completely depressed me. Time after time, I heard how 'our Michelle hadn't lost any weight because she still enjoyed raiding the bicky jar and eating her favourite chocolate digestives'. The conclusion stared me in the face: diets were boring and restrictive, and so my weight loss was doomed if I continued trying to comply with a menu plan that made me feel as if I was in a straitjacket. I decided to leave my slimming club because for me, the only thin thing there was, was the stark lack of available motivation. Don't get me wrong, there are some excellent ones out there, but much depends on the motivational style of the club leader. Unfortunately, the leaders I had could not have encouraged someone dying from thirst to drink the coldest bottle of mineral water in the fridge.

I guess many of you also face similar challenges and struggles to the ones I have had to overcome. On many occasions, I would make excuses not to go out with friends because I felt too fat and ugly. Often, I would feel guilty ordering a fatty dessert off the menu as people looked on thinking, as many do, that I could do without the pudding because, well, I looked rather like one myself. It all began to spiral out of control as the depression kicked in and I stayed put in the house. And yes, you've guessed it, this triggered a cycle of emotional eating. It was simple: I felt bad about myself so I would eat more, and, of course, the first signs of stress made me run to the freezer for ice cream, which incidentally, I mixed with chocolate cookies. Emotional eating made me fatter and at this point, my stomach was so big I was unable to see the floor below. It wasn't as though I didn't know what to eat to become slimmer. For me, the 'what to eat' part has always been common sense and to be honest, I think the majority would be in agreement with me. There are brigades of middle-class nutritionists out there who always make me cringe because they don't live in the real world. They advise the nation on the latest and best super foods to eat, emphasising how they can be used to conquer any health problem. Fortunately, I have managed to find a few who do live in the real world, and who don't waste their energy on blaming food manufacturers, or treat people like idiots.

Okay, rant over! The missing ingredient for me personally was the control I had over food and the inability to make a lifestyle change conducive to weight loss and, equally important, the ability to maintain a healthy weight through sensible eating and exercise. Back then, food controlled me. The chocolate muffin would speak out to me, saying, 'eat me – go on, eat me!' Yes, in those days, food was the boss and I was the subordinate who carried out all its instructions, rarely questioning what I was doing. Fortunately, through a range of practical techniques that I will be sharing with you in this book, I managed to change my situation and regain self-control.

As time passed, enough was enough, I realised that only I could do something about losing weight, not my family, friends or GP. Eventually I managed to remove the unwanted weight, not by surgery, and not by restrictive diets, but entirely through adopting a new lifestyle, which made weight loss both bearable – and wait for it, enjoyable. It wasn't hard any more. I developed a plan of secrets that I will share with you, as we go through this book together. Over the last few years, I have supported thousands of people to move from a world of fat into a world of slim and my mission to help more and more people be the person they really want to be came together in the hit Sky1 and Sky Living TV show, *Fat Families*.

I want you to keep this book with you at all times because I understand the struggles and the negative emotions that being overweight brings. From these pages, I want to bring you hope, but I also want you to understand that at times I will be direct. Many of you will already be familiar with my straight-talking style. The reason for this is that if I allow you to make excuses, nothing will change in your life and you will not lose the weight that you want to. You will stay fat and miserable, with fragile self-esteem just as I had. I will be honest with you and offer you practical tools to lose the weight and also to keep that weight off, but do understand, from the word go, that I cannot do it for you. If I had a magical pill to make people lose weight, I would be a billionaire – but I don't and so it's important you realise that you, and only you, can do it. Take this book everywhere with you. Keep it somewhere safe, never lend it out, and treat it as your very own 'weight loss bible'. It will be a friend to inspire, and it will speak directly to you, so that you have faith in yourself. If you're ever feeling as though you are tempted to fail, grab hold of this book, read one of the secrets, and let it be your source of inspiration.

Remember, I'm on your side. Now let's get to work. For more information on the services I offer, visit www.thestevemillerplan.com. Please note that I have changed the names of people in the book to ensure confidentiality is observed.

SECRET 1

TAKE ON THE 'R' WORD

According to the NHS Information Centre, in 2009 almost a quarter of adults (22 per cent of men and 24 per cent of women aged 16 or over) in England were classified as obese. Furthermore, a greater proportion of men than women (44 per cent compared with 33 per cent) in England were classified as overweight. Yes, we are also the fattest nation in Europe and the number continues to rise. It's no wonder that I now find myself being contacted by the Minister for Public Health for ideas on how to deactivate the obesity time bomb that's about to explode. The government has pumped out a lot of health education campaigns recently, with many aimed at people eating sensibly and taking regular exercise.

Latest findings show that 25 per cent of boys aged between 2 and 19 are overweight or obese, which rises to a staggering 33 per cent for girls. Initiative after initiative continues to fail. That's exactly why I continue to fight to encourage the ever-growing nation of obese inhabitants to take responsibility for their minds and bodies, and get on with weight loss themselves. You may have seen in the media that I hold some strong views on how we need to get a grip and lose the weight for ourselves. It would also seem that the majority agree with me, however, politicians seem unable to act on my advice for fear of losing votes. Sadly, political correctness is now so rife in the UK that it has contributed to making the nation even fatter.

DO IT FOR YOURSELF

It may not be a popular thing to say, but in my view, the British continue to fail in taking responsibility for their own weight. If there's one thing we are really good at, then it has to be making excuses for being too fat. If you were to ask me is it the fault of the food manufacturers, the demands on our time or friends and family, for putting pressure on us, my answer would be a definite no. To say yes would achieve one thing – it would keep you fat, and that would not be fair on you. Of course, it would be more politically correct to campaign for food manufacturers to stop putting so much sugar and fats in the food they make, or encourage the government to pass legislation to ban fast food, chocolate bars, cakes and muffins, but that would bring about a nanny culture that would harm the economy and take away the pleasure factor for those people who can enjoy a treat. Pleasure, I hear you shout!

Well, this is where you may be surprised because I adore a bit of junk food every now and then. Most weeks I have a bottle of wine, a take-away, a cake and a chocolate bar! That's because restrictive diets fail, and flexible ones do not. In fact, if I were told never to eat junk food again, I would probably decide to be fat. Come on, would you really want to live life without an ice cream, a chip butty or a cake? The good news is that living by my ABC, you will still be able to enjoy these treats, week after week. My 80–20 rule allows you to avoid rigidity, making eating a pleasure. I hope that brings a sigh of relief. Yes, 80 per cent of the time you will eat healthily, and 20 per cent of the time you will enjoy a bit of junk food as a treat – and quite right, too!

REFRAME YOUR THINKING

So, when was the last time you heard someone explain to you that weight loss is easy? Indeed, when was the last time an overweight friend explained that they were really looking forward to losing weight? At this point, you are probably thinking that I've gone completely cuckoo and lost the plot. Yes, I guess the answer to these questions is either never, or rarely. As a society we have built a culture around weight loss that pigeonholes it as something that's a massive challenge and a chore. At best, it's difficult and at worst, it's a nightmare! I did the same for many years until I decided to look at how I was thinking about my own weight loss. The penny dropped when I recognised that I was preventing myself from losing the weight by the power of my own thought: I had seen weight loss as an immense battle for far too long. The first step was to reframe my thinking; to keep on telling myself every day that losing weight was hard, difficult, a pain and a struggle would do one thing – keep me fat.

NEW THOUGHTS, NEW BODY

From today, I want you to change the way you think about your weight-loss journey. Forget thinking weight loss is going to bring you pain, introduce difficulties and become an uphill struggle. Instead, see it as something that's exciting, a pleasure, something that's going to be like a trip you have always wanted to do, but never been able to afford. See your weight loss trip as a shared journey, as one you are taking with me. I'll be your constant friend and support. We may have the odd time when you fall down along the way, but I'll be there to pick you up because that's what friends do and I know that we both want the same outcome for you.

Listen out to those around you who moan and groan about how difficult it is to lose weight, and who don't feel guilty for sharing their cynical opinions with others. In fact, make it clear to them that you disagree and that for you, successful weight loss is as good as winning the lottery – well, almost! Of course, these people will think you've gone slightly bonkers and need to see a psychiatrist for sharing such sound advice. However, it will be *you* who best understands because you will experience at first hand that the UK has an ingrained culture, one that makes most people perceive the whole experience of weight loss as a big mountain to climb, and one that you'll undoubtedly fall off and always find impossible to climb. For you, the first big step has been taken. You are now seeing weight loss as something that's your passion, your pleasure and of course, your priority. So, I'll help you get your crampons on, provide you with the ropes, show you how to use the ice axe and give you plenty of oxygen so that we can climb any weight-loss mountain together!

BUST THE EXCUSES

Excuses are often what keeps people fat. I know it isn't always popular to say, but as human beings we are very good at conjuring them up and blaming others for the way we are. Now I want to encourage you to be completely honest with yourself and bury all the excuses you've used over the years for not losing the weight. I know myself because I used to use many excuses and I was great at blaming others for the size I'd become. No one was putting the food into my mouth except me and I was the one who suffered from can't-be-bothered-itis! Fortunately, the day came when I realised I had to do it for myself. I thought through all the excuses I was making and decided to bury them for good. From now on, it was me, and me alone, who could – and *would* – do something about it. I want you to feel the same.

Typical excuses may include:

- It's harder as you get older.
- It's hard with children because I pick at their leftovers.
- I don't know why I'm so fat because I hardly eat anything.
- It's too expensive to eat healthily these days.
- We've always been fat in our family so I guess there's nothing I can do.
- I don't have time to do any exercise.
- I get so stressed and food makes me feel better.
- I work full time and with a family, I just don't have time to eat healthy foods.
- I eat the same as Jean next door, but she's as thin as a rake.

- I just like food and eating it. It's good for you, anyway.
- I'm just one of those people who puts weight on easily.
- Diets are boring and let's face it who wants to live on salad?

Do any of the above ring bells with you? Whenever I'm working with clients, I always begin by agreeing from the outset that excuses will be instantly ditched. If we allow excuses into our sessions we simply let the fat win and nothing will change. Try writing down the excuses you often make and then underneath write a response to bust them. For example, one of my excuses used to be that I liked junk food too much. Now my response to that is that I can enjoy a little junk food without having to deny myself. I also used to blame the food for being so bloody tasty for making me fat! My response now is that no one else makes me eat it, healthy food can be cheaper than ready meals and it's more widely available than ever before. Plus, healthy food can be just as tasty as junk food. As you work your way through this book, I'll continue to offer you more tools and advice to help you blow all the excuses you have away. We don't do excuses anymore, so just forget them!

MANIFEST IT

As you move forward in your quest to shed the pounds, I want you to live life as though you have already lost the weight. You may have heard of the term 'manifesting expectation'. Well, there's a lot of science around the subject of manifestation, which to some is a reality but to others is completely bonkers. No matter how you look at it, though, there can be no doubt that if you expect and believe something will happen, it's more likely to do so.

Right now, just take a few moments to imagine you have already lost the weight and that you now live life at your ideal weight. Perhaps close your eyes as you do so and pay attention to how good it feels. As you wake each day, I want you to live life as though you are already slim. Combine this with the other techniques I describe in the book and you'll be surprised at how much it helps. Live life from this moment accepting personal responsibility for your weight and let excuses dissolve so that you're always in the zone of ultimate success – a weight-loss success.

Katherine's story

Katherine came to see me recently complaining she was fed up of being fat, that the world only accepted, as she put it, 'thin people' and that life was mean to those who were overweight. But Katherine also had every excuse in the cookbook and blamed food manufacturers, her mother, her age and lack of time for her weight. If I'd wanted to write a book on how not to lose weight that day, Katherine would have provided solid content. She thought I had a magic pill and if I waved a magic wand as she took it, it would help her to wake up six stone lighter.

As she sat in my consulting room, I allowed her to ramble on for around 20 minutes before asking her what she actually wanted. 'To make me slimmer, of course!' she barked. When I asked her how I was to do that, she yelled, 'Well, you do it for everyone, don't you?' Sitting there, with a mixture of emotions, I politely explained that actually my clients do it for themselves. With a confused look on her face, the penny finally started to drop. Katherine was beginning to realise that she had to take some responsibility for being overweight and that the excuses she was using would just keep her fat.

During that first session, we talked through all the excuses she was using and one by one, we agreed to bin them. I explained to Katherine that excuses were the cancer of weight loss and to carry them forward would mean she would stay fat — and probably get fatter. Having written down all her excuses, Katherine decided to tear them all up and make a clean start, perceiving the route to weight loss as one of personal responsibility. I explained to her that if she was unwilling to accept responsibility, I would not be willing to see her again as the whole process would be a waste of her time — and mine. That day kick-started a new beginning for Katherine. She acknowledged that blaming the food manufacturers, fast food outlets and other people would not get her anywhere close to the weight she wanted to be. As we moved forward, she turned out to be one of the most fun clients I have ever worked with. We would laugh and make weight loss an exciting pleasure rather than a chore. With responsibility owned and excuses ditched, Katherine went on to lose three stone. She continues to shed more unwanted weight.

David's story

In early 2008, I had an urgent request from a new a client called David. He explained that his weight had spiralled out of control and that he was, as he put it, 'at his wits' end'. I agreed to see him and we set the date for our first session. At 35, David wanted to lose weight so that he stood more of a chance of finding a partner and to improve his career prospects, too. Before meeting David, he sounded convincing and from our telephone conversation he seemed to have a good idea about what he needed to do to lose weight. How wrong I was! When David arrived, he offered me a half-hearted handshake and looked angry and fed up. Thinking it might be nerves, I invited him to sit down and we started to chat. David suddenly went into a sermon on how he had tried all the diets out there and had seen several weight-loss specialists, but *they* had failed to help him lose weight. In his mind, it was all about how other people had failed him and the fact that *they* had been useless. Where have I heard this before? I pondered as I continued to listen to him blaming others for his downfall.

Around 30 minutes passed by until I decided to interrupt him and kindly asked why *he* had failed. Shocked and horrified, his jaw nearly hit the floor — no one had ever spoken to him like that before. '*Me*, failed?' he asked. 'Yes, *you*,' I replied. No one had ever challenged his thought processes before and for a moment he paused and looked at me, not really knowing what to say. I then went on to tell David that all he'd done was blame other people and call them failures, but he'd forgotten to include himself.

Following this, I explained to him that if all he was going to do was blame others and call them failures, he wouldn't move forward and working together would be an absolute waste of time. I asked him to think about the advice he had previously been given — which, to be fair, sounded reasonable, with the exception of a few diets that were restrictive in nature. As our conversation continued, David began to realise that he had to look at himself and his reactions closely. Blaming others would leave him lame, he wouldn't be able to move forward and this would ultimately keep him fat.

As the message sunk in, he acknowledged I had a point and agreed to move forward and accept his responsibility to losing weight. It was David's acceptance of responsibility that was his catalyst to lose weight and in doing so he went on to drop several stone. I am sure he reflects on that message each time he hears people blaming others for their weight. Ultimately, David realised that only he could lose weight for himself; saying that others failed him was actually the perfect excuse and ultimately, one that would have kept him fat.

SECRET 2

FIND YOUR MOTIVATION

Motivation is what drives your weight loss. It's the powerhouse of effective long-lasting weight loss; without it, you are doomed. It's all very well having an eating plan and an exercise regime in place, and you telling yourself that you have to do it, but without motivation it's likely you will fall at the first hurdle. In this chapter, I will offer you a range of practical strategies to help ensure your motivation remains high at all times. The vast majority of people start their weight-loss journey with motivation brimming over the top, only to find after a couple of weeks that it has all dried up. That's why it's essential you have in your weight-loss cupboard a number of tools that will help ensure your motivation has the legs to stay the distance with you.

There are two types of motivation. First, you have 'pull' style motivation. In other words, this style of motivation is the things you are pulled towards, such as seeing yourself slip into that new dress, or being able to play with the kids in the park. The other style of motivation is the opposite to pull, and yes, it's called 'push' style motivation. This is when you are motivated by the negative consequences of being overweight, such as having health problems or getting so fat that you feel completely unattractive. The secret here is to use a combination of both pull and push styles in your weight-loss journey to motivate you into losing weight. For the best possible results, use a combination of the tools that I offer you, and use them at different times over the course of your journey.

PULL STYLE MOTIVATORS
Pin up the outfit
If your motivation to lose weight is to slip into a special outfit that you've had your eye on for a while, then go out and buy it today. Take pleasure as you visit your favourite store, knowing that before long you will be celebrating as you slip into that sexy frock, or the tight pair of jeans that really shows off your rear. When you return home, take out the outfit, hold it up and then chose somewhere to hang it up where it's visible so that you see it frequently. As you look at it, imagine how good you'll feel when you wear it out and the compliments you will receive from the people around you. If it helps, take a picture of it on your phone so that you can quickly glance at it if ever you are tempted to consume too much junk food or alcohol. This will help you stay on course.

Pin up the success chart
Nothing can be more satisfying than seeing how your success is progressing. Design a large poster to represent

how many pounds you need to lose. For example, if you have 27kg (60lb) to lose, you could draw sixty blocks of lard. As each pound drops, rub out a block of lard. This will not only help you feel satisfied, but form a good visual motivator, too. However, if you put a pound back on, then I'm afraid you have to redraw the block of lard. Follow my advice from now on and I promise you it won't come to that, though.

Wallpaper with affirmations

Like things visual? You can also write down a number of positive affirmations and put them in a place where you will see them during the day. If this suits you, then the 'see and feel' motivational tool will work well, too. Use brightly coloured card and write your affirmations in black block capitals. As you see them each day, focus on the words and let those words drift into your mind and become deeply embedded. Typical places to put them can include: on the fridge, on food cupboards, on the bathroom mirror, in your purse or wallet, on the back of the front door and even above the mirror in your lounge! Affirmations should be short and to the point so they are easily absorbed into your mind. Some examples include:

- 'I am a successful slimmer.'
- 'I am proud to be in control of food.'
- 'I melt the lard every day.'
- 'I feel brilliant about my new life.'
- 'I'm excited about my new dress.'
- 'I see myself sexier and slimmer.'
- 'I enjoy my new health.'

- 'I am the boss of food.'
- 'I know losing weight is easy.'
- 'I hear myself being so much more confident.'
- 'I see a new me every day.'
- 'I feel so focused and excited about losing weight each day.'
- 'I love to hear the compliments others say.'
- 'I feel so in control of my life and food.'

The list can go on. However, a word of caution: avoid using the word 'not' in your affirmations as this can have the reverse affect. For example, if I were to say to you, 'do not think of a chocolate biscuit', invariably you will do just that and picture your favourite chocolate digestive! Always keep the affirmations positive.

Develop a flirt plan and enjoy it!

Well, it has to be said, there's nothing like a good old flirt! And, as they say, window-shopping is absolutely fine if you are in a relationship. I remember the newfound attention I was showered with after I lost all my weight and boy, oh boy, did it make me feel great! Whether you like it or not, we judge people initially on the way they look. And yes, men are initially more drawn to what they see, rather than what they hear and do: judging a book by its cover. So, if your motivation is about feeling better about your image and being attractive to others, there is nothing wrong with a bit of gentle flirting. Let's face it, it's fun and it doesn't half make you feel good if the flirting is reciprocated. If flirting more as the weight drops off is one of your motivators, let me share a few tips:

- Give three different verbal or non-verbal signals. When you give the first signal the other person is going to check to see if it's really them that you are checking out. However, the second time they know it's them and believe me, they will be pleased! The third time you can perhaps make small talk, such as explaining how you like what he or she is wearing, or express interest by asking them over and informing them that you recognise their face. As you start chatting, move away from the crowd a little. The person you're having the flirt with doesn't want to feel you will reject them in front of others, so create a bit of space. If you go out with a friend, then do separate every so often or take a breather from talking because people won't want to risk your disapproval by interrupting you.

- Treating people gently is also very important. If someone flirts with you and you are not interested in him or her, be kind. Avoid raising your eyes disapprovingly, or laughing as that person walks away. Be realistic and not mean because if you do this, you are limiting your chances of other people approaching you.

- With your body shrinking day by day, monitor your body language as you flirt so that it looks confident. Sit and stand tall. It really is amazing how much more confident you will appear if you do this. Your outward presence increases and others will see you as someone they respect and would actually like to talk to. The same goes with your eyes; smile with them, as well as with your mouth. And above all, as you do so, remind

15

yourself how losing weight is turning you into a sex magnet.

- If you fancy playing a game, walk through a group of women or men and see which of them is checking you out. Remember, even if it's just one or two, enjoy! The weight is dropping and you are becoming irresistible. Before long, it will be the whole crowd who can't keep their eyes off you.
- As the weight drops off, there's nothing wrong with making yourself more irresistible. Consider wearing new make-up, showing a little flesh, wearing different accessories, or even getting yourself a completely new hairdo.

Be a role model to your children

There's no doubt that as your lifestyle changes and you eat less, eat more healthily and become more active, the example you set to your children will be excellent and will motivate you even further. It's a fact that there is a direct relationship between fat parents and fat kids. This isn't a genetic inevitability, but one of pure lifestyle habit that parents pass on to their offspring. If a child constantly sees his parents slouching on the sofa and packing in piles of junk food then, and I'm sure you will agree, it's common sense that he will do just the same. And it's logical to assume that the parents are overfeeding their kids on piles and piles of junk food, and that they too will become fat. It's rightly said that underfeeding kids is child cruelty, but I also believe overfeeding kids is just the same. This may sound like a push style of motivation, but I want us to make it a pull style. In other words, a motivation that will excite you, knowing your children are becoming fitter, healthier and less likely to suffer health problems because you are leading the way for them to follow.

Being a role model to your kids is something you can be truly proud of. You can stand at the school gate knowing other children aren't looking at you and thinking, 'That's little Tommy's mum, I'm not surprised he's so fat!' Or take sports day as another example, when parents can go and see their children take part and share in the fun and pride of them being active. The reality is that embarrassment kicks in for the kids whose parents struggle to fit on one seat, or always come last in the parents' race being a complete chunk. Believe me, this is the real world, and I want you to let this real world motivate you into becoming the best possible role model. Getting the whole family involved in your weight loss can be great fun, so consider some of the following ideas:

- Make lists with the kids to go shopping using the 80–20 rule, which I discuss in more detail later in this book (page 67).
- Cook healthy food with your children: encourage them to roll up their sleeves and really get stuck in!
- Explain to them that as soon as you lose a certain amount of weight that you will be celebrating by taking everyone on a day out.
- Take up a family sport that you can all participate in together. Keep it simple, such as a weekly swim, cycling, trekking or if the children are older, try Zumba classes.
- Ask the kids to develop a weekly menu plan using the 80–20 rule. Explain that a prize will be given for the best weekly plan.

- Plan a night-time walk in the summer (take a route that's safe and exciting). Kids love the adventure of this.
- Like the gym? Why not join as a family if your kids are old enough? These days, there are some great rates to be had for family gym memberships.
- Take up hobbies and interests as a family: remember, a bored mind becomes a hungry one. Perhaps start doing something different, such as archery or kite surfing.
- Share your newfound knowledge about portion control, motivation, the 80–20 rule of eating and all the motivational tips that you are picking up with the kids.

Have treats along the way

If you do well, you deserve a reward – and why not? There was a time when I would have said never reward with food or alcohol, but I was wrong. Of course, I'm not suggesting you run to the local Indian and have a large curry and a whole bottle of wine because you've lost a pound – that would be ludicrous. What I encourage you to do is include some treats in line with my 80–20 philosophy along the way. An alternative would be to treat yourself to a new outfit, perfume or even a bunch of flowers to celebrate your achievement. If you are losing weight as a family, then bring in family treats, such as a day out at a theme park, a trip to the cinema or tenpin bowling.

Do a daily success report

Logging your daily achievement can be a productive way to reinforce positive actions as you progress. In working together, I want you to focus your thoughts and the words you speak on positive ideas. Negative thoughts and words will do nothing but keep you fat, so at the end of the day, writing down your thoughts on how well you have done can really help motivate you in the days that follow. Of course, I'm not suggesting there will be no issues or rocky patches along the way – after all, as a human being you are fallible. However, what I would direct you to do is to write down solutions to some of the bumps and traps you might encounter in your daily report instead of just listing the problems. Once again, remember problems and excuses are the enemy and keep you fat. Use a logbook to write down your successes using the following framework:

- Success with food, including the type of food you ate during the day based on the 80–20 rule of eating. Include successes in portion control.
- No matter how small, success in doing some exercise: examples might include getting up at 7am and doing half an hour's brisk walk before getting ready for work.
- Success in your positive attitude, such as remembering to tell yourself that weight loss is exciting and actually easy.
- Dealing with aspects of your life that have made you fat, such as ditching so-called friends who de-motivate and drain you, and taking up hobbies and interests to alleviate boredom.
- Successes using the mind programming tools I explain later in this book (see page 155).

This is not an exhaustive list. Feel free to write anything in your daily success report that will help to keep your motivation sky-high.

Change your body language

This is one of the practical things I did when my own fat began to melt away. As the weight drops off, I want you to change the way you use your body language. I want you to deliberately act as if you are confident, which will be so much easier to do now you are losing the weight. As you do this, you will not only project more positivity, but you will also feel so much better in yourself. It's a proven fact that changing our physiology also changes our mood and the way we feel about ourselves. This will motivate you to go on, lose more weight *and* keep it off. Examples may include:

- Walking tall with a neat, upright posture.
- Applying gestures to emphasise words, making your communication more colourful.
- Using eye contact, which illustrates a new, confident you.
- Sitting upright and alert at your desk or in meetings.

PUSH STYLE MOTIVATORS
Health in jeopardy means you could die early

Now I don't have to tell many of you that being too fat also brings the likelihood of illness (and most probably, an early death), but for many this is not a concern for today. However, you may not have sat down and really thought about each of the potential health consequences of doing nothing about your weight. If health is your motivator, it's time to consider the impact of being overweight.

You may have recently seen in the press that Type 2 diabetes is a disease in which blood sugar levels are above normal. Worryingly, high blood sugar is a major cause of coronary heart disease, kidney disease, stroke, amputation and blindness. Type 2 diabetes is often associated with obesity and a significant proportion of people with this condition are overweight. It's thought that being overweight causes cells in the body to change, making them resistant to the hormone insulin. Insulin carries sugar from blood to the cells, where it is used for energy. When a person is insulin resistant, blood sugar cannot be taken up by the cells, resulting in high blood sugar. You can definitely reduce your risk of developing Type 2 diabetes by losing weight and increasing the amount of exercise you do.

If you already have Type 2 diabetes, losing weight and becoming more physically active can help you control your blood sugar levels and prevent or delay complications. Losing weight and exercising more may also allow you to reduce the amount of diabetes medication you take. You can reverse the condition and be very proud that you have done it!

Among those who are too fat, coronary heart disease and strokes are frequent killers. Coronary heart disease means the heart and circulation of blood do not function normally. Usually, the arteries have become hardened and narrowed. If you have coronary heart disease, you may suffer a heart attack, congestive heart failure, sudden cardiac death, angina or abnormal heart rhythm. In a heart attack, the flow of blood and oxygen to the heart is disrupted, damaging portions of the heart muscle. During a stroke, blood and oxygen do not flow normally to the brain, which can cause paralysis or even death. People who are overweight are more likely to develop high blood pressure, hard fats in the blood and high levels of bad cholesterol. These are all increased risk factors for heart disease and a stroke. The good news is that losing 5–10 per cent of your weight can lower the chances of you developing coronary heart disease or having a stroke. Weight loss can also reduce blood pressure and cholesterol levels, as well as improving your heart function and blood flow.

One of the health risks that often we don't want to mention but you really must be aware of if you are overweight is cancer. It occurs when cells in one part of the body, such as the colon, grow abnormally or out of control. Sometimes the cancerous cells spread to other parts of the body, such as the liver, the lungs or the brain, too. Being overweight can increase your risk of developing several types of cancer, including cancer of the colon, oesophagus and kidney. Gaining weight during adult life increases the risk of getting several of these cancers, even if the weight gain does not result in you being overweight or obese. Eating better and improving your physical activity may prevent a rise in the risk of cancer.

Sleep apnoea is a disorder that happens when a person stops breathing for short periods during the night. It is much more common in those who are fat. The reason for this is that the person who is overweight may have more fat around his or her neck, which makes the airway smaller. This smaller airway can make breathing difficult and trigger very loud snoring, or cause that person to stop breathing altogether. Weight loss will normally improve sleep apnoea because it decreases the size of the neck.

Osteoarthritis is a joint disorder that causes the joint bone and cartilage to wear away. It commonly affects the joints in the knees, hips and lower back and this can cause a lot of pain. Being overweight may place extra pressure on the joints and cartilage causing them to wear away prematurely. Research indicates that losing at least 5 per cent of your body weight may decrease stress on the knees, hips and lower back.

Gallbladder disease includes gallstones and inflammation or infection of the gallbladder. Gallstones are mostly made up of cholesterol and can cause lots of abdominal pain, especially after eating fatty foods. People who are overweight have a higher risk of developing a gallbladder disease because they may produce more cholesterol, which is the root cause of gallstones. Gradual weight loss of up to 1kg (2lb) a week may lower your risk of developing gallstones.

Fat infiltration in the liver can cause liver disease and this comes about when fat builds up in the liver cells, so causing inflammation and long-term damage to the organ. It can sometimes lead to severe liver damage, cirrhosis or even liver failure. Fatty liver disease is similar to liver damage caused by too much alcohol, but it is not caused by alcohol and can actually occur in those who drink little or no alcohol. People who have diabetes or 'pre-diabetes' (when blood sugar levels are higher than normal but not yet in the diabetic range) are more likely to have fatty liver disease than those without these conditions. People who are overweight are more likely to develop diabetes (see the 'Type 2 diabetes' section, page 21). It is not known why some people who are overweight or diabetic get fatty liver disease while others do not. Losing weight and being physically active will help you control your blood sugar levels. It can also reduce the build-up of fat in your liver and prevent further injury. People with fatty liver disease should avoid drinking alcohol.

Develop a restaurant warning

Do you ever enter a restaurant determined to eat sensibly only to find you end up having a big blow out? You walk out feeling guilty, beat yourself up and feel completely tortured. What I advise is to design yourself a little restaurant warning sign on a postcard and take it along with you. As you enter the restaurant, glance at it and let it be your motivator, the one that stops you ordering fat-feeding dishes and instead turns you straight to the healthy option. Some example warning statements may include:

- If you are FAT, then THINK before ordering.
- Eat FAT, stay FAT.
- STOP and THINK, or be FAT.
- People in this restaurant will think I am FAT and GREEDY if I choose junk food.
- FAT KILLS – Think!
- Eat FAT and you will remain a FATTY!

These may sound a little harsh, but motivation is also about reminding yourself truthfully of the consequences and of course, the truth hurts. I can't apologise for my straight-talking style as I know it works and this may well help if you are a social butterfly who often dines out. Also, if there's nothing on the menu that you think is healthy for you to eat, never be afraid of asking the waiter to offer you something that isn't as loaded with calories as the items you see before you on the menu.

Don't forget that alcohol is also very calorific, and it's easy to consume more when eating out. I should know having been a slave to wine years ago. The wine did nothing but add weight to my belly! A few drinks are OK, but if you are one of those people that starts but can't stop my advice would be to go cold turkey for now, and then slowly begin introducing the odd drink now and then when you are eating out. If your friends try to push you to drink then learn to be more assertive at the dinner table. (See page 56 for details on applying assertive behaviour.)

Observe the daily reality of fat

Bringing the reality of fat to a conscious level will help to motivate you away from that lifestyle. From this moment on, aim to deliberately observe fat people's habits. Notice how many of them continue to eat food as though it's going out of fashion and see how they are often the ones at the front of the queue when the buffet is announced open. Listen to the ridiculous excuses they use, such as 'I'm only having this because I'm not eating tonight'. Of course, we all know that old line! Why do they stay fat then? Let's face it: no one gets fat on fresh air! This is not about being cruel to those who are fat; it's about paying attention to their behaviour and the fat-feeding habits they adopt. Be angry at the habits, not the person and let them motivate you away from a world of fat.

The reality of being fat parents

I'm often asked the question, 'Do fat parents make good parents?' In short, if a parent is fat of course they can still be a good parent. However, if I were asked the question, 'Are fat parents good role models for their child's health?' then the answer would be a solid NO. There's no getting away from the fact that kids look to their parents as role models. For this reason young children begin to copy Mummy and Daddy – and this includes what they eat, the quantity of food they consume and how active they are in their lives. If the parents eat junk food and move like a pair of snails, then it's not surprising that their children eventually become obese. What pains me more is when I see fat kids being taken out by their parents to fast food restaurants to eat burgers, chips, cakes and ice cream. Ultimately, this is a form of childhood cruelty and I believe the majority of people think this way too, even though they might not admit to it. If you are one of those parents, let this message motivate you to turn your bad lifestyle choices into good ones for you and your family.

However, there is nothing wrong with taking the kids out for the odd fast food treat. This is part of the real world, and I would never advocate denying kids a bit of junk food here and there. What is important is to educate them so that they understand that food intake is about balance: 80 per cent healthy and 20 per cent a bit of what you fancy!

Apply tough love

Like millions of others, you may have repeatedly tried to lose weight only to keep slipping down the uphill climb that will eventually lead to the slim you. For most people, this has meant momentarily giving up and turning to chocolate bars for comfort, only to find yourself back where you started and as fat as ever, days later. To help maintain focus, many find that applying tough love works really well in ensuring their journey never deviates from the weight-loss ascent. In reality, this may mean giving yourself a kick up the backside when you are tempted to dive into too many bowls of crisps, drink too much alcohol, or not get your bum out of bed for a brisk walk. Yes, at times you have to be tough on yourself because tea, biscuits and tissues to wipe the tears (moping around!) often keep people fat.

Whenever you feel your attitude changing, and you begin to forget all those positive thoughts, or excuses start creeping into your head, apply a dollop of tough love. Tell yourself to stop moaning and get on with it! Be as tough on yourself as you can be, especially if this motivates you to get on with the job.

When working with my own clients, I simply refuse to grant them permission to spurt out a million and one excuses as to why they haven't lost weight and done as we agreed. Fortunately, they know only too well that I won't accept their excuses, meaning they get the results they deserve: it's all about tough love.

Be aware of what most people think

If your motivation is to avoid others judging you, then this motivator is definitely for you. You probably know by now that I refuse to wrap it up because that would not be fair on you. Nor will I succumb to political correctness because that just keeps you fat. At the end of the day, we both want a weight-loss result for you and so honesty really is the best policy. There are many things people think when they see a fat person: most are very negative whether this is right or wrong, it's never going to change. I'm not saying this is fair, but it's true that most people dread the thought of a fat person sitting next to them on a plane, in the cinema or at the theatre. And typical judgements include others believing that fat people are lazy and lack any sense of responsibility. I know it hurts, but I want to encourage you to let this motivate you away from being thought of in that way: there *is* something you can do about it and that's the wonderful thing.

SECRET 3

BE IN CONTROL OF FOOD

Over the years, the opportunity to eat junk food has become much easier due to its affordability. I remember the days when fish and chips were a real treat. Nowadays, it's relatively easy to buy them a few times a week. Not only that, but fatty, sugary foods are often on special offer in supermarkets and it doesn't break the bank to buy profiteroles, mini donuts, tubs of ice cream and chocolate bars. We are effectively spoilt for choice, especially given the fact that you can buy a pack full of treats for £1, or take advantage of the numerous buy one, get one free deals that we see everywhere. This is one of the reasons why food has gained the upper hand over the years, taking control of you rather than *you* taking control of it. In short, so many people have become slaves to food. It's become the champ and celebrates a victory every time you buy into all the unhealthy items in store because your mind is conditioned to believe it pulls the strings. Food has tempted you, and for no fault of your own, you gave in to this temptation by eating it – and eating too much of it, too.

In other words, the control food has is superior because your subconscious mind has become programmed to eat rubbish food, and lots of it. Now I'm all for eating a bit of junk but when junk is in the majority, it becomes a different story. It turns you into a junk product, one that gets caught in a spiral of eating to feel good, feeling bad about yourself and then eating some more just to feel good again.

It's when you take the control back that your eating patterns will be healthier; helping you to slim down to the person you deserve to be. In this chapter, I offer you a number of strategies to help you regain control. Try them all, and then select the ones that work best for you.

THE GREEN CROSS CODE

Over the next coming days, I want you to start experiencing food using the Green Cross Code: stop, look and listen. However, in this instance you will be using the code in the context of food control. This technique has helped thousands of my clients bring back the control they have over food, so that they eat less and eat better:

- *Stop:* Before you decide to eat, start making a conscious effort to stop and think about what you're about to do. This also includes stopping as soon as you see the food in front of you, which is probably yelling, 'eat me, eat me!' As you look at the food, deliberately stop yourself from reaching out to it. The reality is the food wants you to grab it and put it straight in your mouth without even thinking. Because you have done this for so long, it's natural to get in there and munch on whatever you see but from now on, I want you to STOP first.

- *Look:* Now that you've stopped, take a good look at what's in front of you. Is it healthy, or is it food that will do nothing for your waistline other than make you fat? LOOK at what you see. Using your commonsense and the advice given in this book, ask yourself: do you see food that contains a lot of fat and a high calorific content, or food that is low in fat and low in calories? At this point, keep your hands by your side and silently begin to congratulate yourself on what you are doing. At this point, it really is important to slow down and say 'well done' to yourself as your ability to control the food becomes much stronger.
- *Listen:* Having stopped and looked at the food, it's now time to LISTEN to your inner voice. The best way to do this is by asking yourself three key questions: What will this do for me? What can I do differently? What does it feel like, knowing I have power over it?

If you decided that you don't want the food after all, promptly dispose of it and turn your back on it. Once again, congratulate yourself and be sure to smile! Then select a healthy option and as you eat it slowly, congratulate yourself again and affirm mentally that you are in control of the food. Assert the control you have over food in your mind as many times as possible, as this will help you to develop a new and positive habit.

Use the Green Cross Code method of food control in as many situations as possible, especially where temptation is present, such as Christmas parties, weddings, birthdays and all those social gatherings where you are likely to face loads of calorie-laden foods, and where often you can eat as much as you like.

MAINTAIN AN ACTIVE MIND

Have you ever noticed that you eat when you are bored? Isn't it easy to grab hold of some crisps and dips, or sweets and eat to occupy the mind? For many people, weight gain is often the result of picking at food. I would advise you to plan your time carefully in between meals, making sure that your brain is engaged so you are mentally busy. In between your three meals a day, plan things to do, such as reading, writing, walking, or focusing on your work. Try and do something where your full concentration is away from food and focused instead on what you are doing. Avoid sitting around doing nothing because your mind may soon begin to wander onto the topic of the food in your fridge. It is amazing how much snacking is done when the mind is bored. People aren't often aware of how much they snack on especially when playing computer games or watching TV, so do bear this in mind too! Remember the saying, 'little pickers wear big knickers'? Stay busy so yours become smaller!

Read the script

I have designed the following script for you to read daily to help your control over food become solid. If you feel this works for you, I would recommend you read it for 21 days. The reason I say 21 days is because it normally takes around three weeks for a new habit to be formed. In other words, what you read will gradually become embedded in your mind, helping you to automatically be in control of food. Simply sit in a comfortable seat where you won't be interrupted and allow the words to drift into your mind, bit by bit. You will also notice that I use pauses between each statement because I want you to take your time. This is to help the suggestions in my script sink deeper into your mind, helping the new habit of control over food to become firmly embedded:

'As you sit reading this [PAUSE] I want you to know that everything I say to you [PAUSE] is for your benefit [PAUSE] so that you become more and more in control of food [PAUSE] because you *deserve* to be in control of food [PAUSE], and I want you to know that as you read this [PAUSE] your full mental concentration is focused on allowing all the things I say to you [PAUSE] for your benefit [PAUSE], so that [PAUSE] over the days that follow [PAUSE] your control over food becomes so much stronger [PAUSE] so much more natural [PAUSE] and [PAUSE] it is completely understandable that in the past food had the upper hand [PAUSE] because in the past you had allowed it to become the boss [PAUSE] the gaffer [PAUSE] the manager of you [PAUSE] and that wasn't your fault [PAUSE], you weren't to blame [PAUSE] it is just that in the past food decided it would lead the way [PAUSE] and back then, you had accepted it would be that way [PAUSE] so there is no need to feel guilty [PAUSE] no need to blame yourself [PAUSE] because right now, you have decided that it's time for a change [PAUSE] time to do something new [PAUSE] something exciting [PAUSE].

'As you read this I want you to smile [PAUSE]. You can smile because I want you to know that right now you are taking back the control [PAUSE] things are changing radically [PAUSE] I suppose it's a bit like a promotion for you [PAUSE], promoted to a position that gives you leadership and control over food [PAUSE] and you deserve it, and [PAUSE] as you read this, I am suggesting deep into your mind that you [PAUSE] yes, *you* [PAUSE], are in control [PAUSE] in control of your choice over food [PAUSE]. More and more, *you* have the ability [PAUSE] to think [PAUSE] and decide for yourself what and how much food you will eat [PAUSE].

'And in the course of selecting what food you will eat [PAUSE], you notice that your choice is more calculated [PAUSE], it is more guided to what you want to eat [PAUSE], all for your benefit [PAUSE] and because you want to slim [PAUSE], slim down into being the person you really want to be [PAUSE]. It is not surprising that you choose healthy foods [PAUSE]. You choose healthy foods because you are now in control [PAUSE] and because you are in control of food, you are feeling so much better about yourself [PAUSE]. These words you hear right now sink into your mind so that the control of food becomes second nature [PAUSE]. In fact, there will be times you don't even think about it because it's automatic [PAUSE].

'Knowing you are now in control of food brings a warm satisfaction with it [PAUSE] and it's not only the choice of food that you control [PAUSE], you are now controlling how much you eat [PAUSE] and because you are in control of how much you eat [PAUSE], you have no desire to binge on food [PAUSE], no desire to binge at all [PAUSE], because for you food control is now about choice and portion [PAUSE] with no desire to binge [PAUSE]. You are pleased to notice that your control is stronger than you ever could imagine [PAUSE]. Food control is with you [PAUSE], deep in your mind [PAUSE], now firmly a part of you [PAUSE], where it will remain for good [PAUSE].'

DIVERSION WITH AVERSION

This is one psychological trick that can work well. It involves creating an aversion to certain foods that you want to eliminate from your life because they are just too fattening. In essence, what you will be doing is programming your mind so that it automatically feels repulsed when it either thinks of, or actually sees particular foods. Recently, I managed to support a client in developing an aversion to jelly sweets.

Lorraine was eating at least two or three packets a day and as they were full of sugar, they were obviously not supporting her weight loss. The aversion technique worked exceptionally well for her as soon as she began to imagine them covered in cottage cheese. Previously, she had explained to me that she had a real distaste for cottage cheese and the thought of jellied sweets mixed with it automatically made her feel sick. If you feel this technique will help you too in gaining control over food you want to stop eating, follow the process described below:

• Close your eyes and relax.
• Mentally count down from ten to one, with each number on every out breath.

- Bring into mind the food that you want to create a dislike for.
- Now bring forward something that for you is distasteful, perhaps even makes you feel a little sick.
- Imagine both fused together. Pay attention to the smell, taste and feelings it stirs.
- Now open your eyes and think about the food responsible for making you gain weight.
- Repeat the process until you notice the aversion is strong.

INSTALL AN AUTOMATIC TRIGGER

Have you ever smelt a perfume which has automatically triggered a memory or an emotional response? Perhaps you might have listened to a piece of music and noticed the automatic emotions it has evoked. The reason this happens is because your subconscious mind has had millions of experiences during your life and with those experiences are attached emotions. So, why am I telling you this? Well, based on this psychological principle (which is known as 'conditioning'), you can also set up an instant sense of control when it comes to food. Let's look at the steps below:

- Sit somewhere comfortable where it is safe to do so, and close your eyes. Drift back to a time when you felt in control. It doesn't matter what the situation was, just drift back into that experience and relive it. See it, hear it and feel it. If you can't think of a time when you felt fully in control, just imagine what it feels like.

- As you sit there intensify the feelings of control. Give those feelings a score out of ten. If they are currently at six, intensify them even more. Intensify so they reach a nine or ten.
- At the point of intensity, squeeze your fist.
- Once you have squeezed your fist, replicate the process all over again. Do this at least six times.
- Now open your eyes and try squeezing your fist.

You may already be feeling a sense of control as you squeeze your fist. If not, don't worry: just keep on using the technique until you do. Over time, your subconscious mind will automatically trigger a sense of control as you squeeze your fist because your inner mind now associates a squeezed fist with a feeling of control. Once established, you can use this technique whenever you feel the need to gain some self-control over food. Simply squeeze your fist and allow the control to help you make sensible decisions over food choices and quantity.

CHAT IT UP

Every single minute of the day, we are engaged in conversation – in fact, it's impossible not to communicate. However, the majority of conversations we have are inside our own mind. We talk to ourselves about how we feel, and we talk to ourselves about other people and the things around us. Naturally, we also do this whenever we see or smell food. Often it's thoughts like, 'Oh, that smells good', or 'I could just eat that'. The academic terminology for this is 'cognition' and our cognitive process is activated as soon as we see food. One of the techniques I have found to benefit my clients is where they hold mental conversations with the food itself. Sounds completely mental? Yes, it probably does, however what you will be doing is taking control of the conversation with the food so you get the upper hand.

Take Joy, who for years had given in to unhealthy food until she finally decided to hold mind conversations with it. In the old days Joy's mind conversation with the food was, 'Hi, you look nice and smell delicious, come into my mouth.' Joy was someone who agreed with the food constantly, and at 114 kilos (18 stone), this was making her pretty miserable. Having coached Joy on mind control with food, she then decided to utilise this particular technique to her advantage. No longer was she in complete agreement with the food when she came into contact with it. Instead, she would mentally inform the food that she was the boss and that she had decided it was not for her. In fact, one of her preferred phrases was, 'Not today, thank you'. Try this technique by following the steps below:

- Look at the food in front of you and then monitor the conversation you are having inside your head.
- If you know the food will make you fat, mentally explain to it that *you* are in control and it's no longer welcome.
- Make it as specific as possible. For example, if you are looking at a tub of ice cream you could mentally say, 'Ice cream, for the last ten years you have had complete control. However, you need to know that the purpose you served in the past is no longer required. Ice cream, I am waving you goodbye because the fat you used to put on my body is no longer a part of who I am. See you

around!' Of course, say this to yourself because if you say it out loud you may well receive some very strange looks!

Use this technique to build your control over certain foods that you have felt addicted to. Over time, it will help you to eat less of them or even say goodbye to them for good.

Martine's story

I met Martine several years ago. She telephoned to book an appointment with me and explained that she couldn't understand why she was eating so much and that it was really getting her down. Her weight had ballooned and she felt that the amount she was eating was just out of control. As I chatted to her, I could feel the desperation in her voice. Martine was in a place where food was the boss, and she felt there was no stopping it from entering her mouth. We agreed to book three sessions to work together with the aim being to help her get back her control over food; we didn't want food to become the enemy but what we did want was for Martine to become in control.

When I met Martine I understood very quickly that for her, eating was often an unconscious process. She explained that she would sit on the sofa and not even be aware of her hand feeding her mouth. As she told me that she would watch films and eat a full bag of chocolates without noticing, she smiled. Martine explained, quite rightly, that for her it was all a 'mind thing'. My goal here was obvious: I had to develop a plan that would help her gain control of her eating habits. That plan was about reprogramming Martine's mind. In other words, I had to help her become more conscious of her eating habits again but also help her bring back some control when eating.

I decided to facilitate a three-stage process. First, by using hypnotherapy, I helped Martine gain control of the part that was responsible for her eating.

For too long she had lost control of her trigger for eating, and therefore just ate and ate without noticing. This helped her become more aware of what she was doing when it came to eating and when we met for her second session, she went on to explain that she was much more conscious of what she was doing and had actually lost 1.5kg (3lb) in a week. She explained that she now noticed specific eating actions, such as her hand moving to eat food. I was thrilled when she reported that she was now making a conscious decision whether to eat the food or not and that she was more aware of her eating habits. This was a first for Martine!

During session two, I carried out another session of hypnotherapy and used direct suggestion. As Martine deeply relaxed, I installed in her mind the idea that she now had no desire to binge and was in control of food. Outside of the hypnotherapy session, we also agreed that she would keep a diary, writing down all her thoughts and emotions during the next week. This would help her become even more conscious of what she was eating.

In our third session, I conducted a final session of hypnotherapy and installed an automatic trigger. The overall process helped Martine gain back the control she had lost over the years. With the control back in her life, she was now in a position to lose weight. Martine's successful weight loss continued and she managed to lose 25 kilos (4 stone). For her, this wasn't about dieting, it was about gaining control over her eating habits. Now, when it comes to food, Martine is aware of every move she makes. Food no longer rules her life.

SECRET 4

PLAN

There isn't a client I have worked with who hasn't mentioned the importance of planning. It's also one of the biggest excuses people use not to lose weight. If I had a pound for every person who has told me they don't have time to eat better and do some exercise, I would be in *The Sunday Times* Rich List. Of course, time is scarce as we live busier lives so it's imperative for us to manage our time so that we can eat less, follow a healthy, balanced diet and get physical as much as possible. In this chapter, I will offer you a number of straightforward time management techniques. You only need to select one because that will automatically help you plan a lifestyle conducive to losing weight and then keeping it off.

THE 'TO DO' LIST

Having a reminder system in the form of a 'to do' list to tell you what and when you need to do it because trying to carry everything in your head is simply a recipe for disaster. Try carrying a pen and paper with you wherever you go, or take a diary to write down the things you need to do. Writing a daily list of tasks that need to be done is an effective way to plan. Refer to it, update it daily and cross things off as you do them. You can also prioritise items that are on the list into important/not important and urgent/non-urgent. Perhaps highlight urgent items to ensure they are the obvious priority. There are many advantages of a 'to do' list including:

- It focuses the mind on important things.
- You become less forgetful as you order your thoughts.
- The 'to do' list immediately reminds you of what you need to do so you save time.
- It helps you decide on priorities and stops you from becoming side-tracked.
- You have a record of what you've done.
- Best of all, you are more in control and you'll feel good as you tick off your achievements.

USING A TIME LOG

A helpful way to eliminate wasted time is through using a time log. To do so, you will need to design a chart for the next seven days divided into half-hour sections, starting at the time you get up and finishing with the time you go to bed. Write down what you did in each half hour of the day for the next seven days (make sure the week you choose is typical). Here is an example:

7.15am: Wake up.

7.30am: Shower and get ready for work.

8am: Eat breakfast and then drive to work.

8.30am: Arrive at work.

10am: Chat with colleagues.

11am: Have a mid-morning break.

11.30am: Work.

12.30pm: Lunch.

1.30pm: Work.

5pm: Finish work and drive home.

5.30pm: Arrive home and chill.

6pm: Make dinner for everyone.

7pm: Watch TV with the family.

8.30pm: Put the kids to bed.

11pm: Go to bed.

At the end of the week examine your time log and ask yourself the following questions:

- Are there any periods when I might have used my time more productively?
- Is there any down time when I could be doing some exercise? For example, can I fit in a session on the Wii Fit between 8.30pm and bedtime?
- Can I delegate any of my tasks to make time for exercise? For example, rotating who prepares dinner.
- Could I get up earlier to do some exercise before work?
- Did I waste any time?

PLANNING AHEAD

A good way to get started is to plan for the week ahead. Write down all the tasks that you need to do in the next week to keep you on your weight-loss course. A key task will be meal planning as this will help you to eat more healthily and by buying only what you need, you will also save money. Plan out your meals and put them into your diary or on a wall planner. Once you have completed the list, write down all your other commitments, such as things to do with the kids, taking the neighbour's dog for a walk, visiting parents and doing the housework, etc.

Once all the tasks are listed in your diary, match things up to make the most of your time. For example, this may include preparing meals for two days or walking the neighbour's dog at the same time as visiting your parents. Planning ahead helps you to work smarter and get a lot more done, so that eating well and exercising more isn't so hard to fit into your busy week.

PROCRASTINATE NO MORE

'Oh, I'll do it tomorrow' or even, 'I can't be bothered to do it now'. Do you ever hear yourself saying this? When you're tired it's so easy to say this, isn't it? I strongly advise you to avoid putting things off for too long because doing this only makes matters worse in the long run. Try to find 15 minutes a day to finish off tasks and complete the ones you had hoped would disappear. Procrastinating only stops you from doing what you really want to do. A good tip is to use down time to get those little jobs done. For example, chop up some vegetables while you wait for the kids to get home from school and take 10 minutes at the end of each day to look over what you need to do tomorrow so you wake up feeling focused. Procrastinating only leaves you feeling like you never have enough time to do what you need to do.

PRIORITISE YOUR ACTIVITIES

Write down your weekly tasks and divide them into three sections. These sections should include:

- Must do.
- Should do.
- Could do.

In the 'must do' section add activities that you feel are critical. This may include meal planning, exercise, mind programming and any other essentials. If you find that too many other activities end up in this section you may need to consider whether you're living by unrealistic expectations. Go on to prioritise what must be done and consider alternative ways of getting tasks done, such as delegating to another member of the family. Each week, write down the tasks suited to each section. Activities you place in the 'must do' and 'should do' sections should always be ticked off whereas those in the 'could do' section are important, but not essential. Always regard the 'could do' category as the luxury section in your time management plan.

SET OBJECTIVES

Objective setting can be a useful motivator. If you are driven by objectives, you can set them as short, medium and long term. When setting goals it's important to make them SMART:

- Specific: To the point and in one sentence.
- Measurable: How you know the goal has been achieved.
- Agreed: Inside your mind you know that you can do it.
- Realistic: You know you have the resources to achieve it.
- Time bound: The date the objective will be achieved.

Let's imagine Dawn wants to lose 19 kilos (3 stone) in weight. To help manage her time she sets short-term (next month) and long-term objectives (at the end of 3–6 months). If today's date is 1 March, her objectives may look like this:

Short-term objectives
- All meal plans to be complete by 5pm each Wednesday.
- Walk for 1 hour per day around the park during March.
- Join a Salsa class by 10 March.
- Lose 1–1.5kg (2–3lb) each week and celebrate with a small reward.
- Begin gentle jogging by 30 March, as agreed with the doctor.

Long-term objectives
- To have lost 12.7kg (2 stone) in weight by 20 July.
- Be a natural Salsa dancer by 30 June.
- Jog non-stop for 1 hour by 10 May.
- Fluently explain the 80–20 rule of meal planning by 10 April.
- Be wearing a size 10 swimsuit by 30 July.

PICK AND MIX

Now take a look at some of my other pick-and-mix time management strategies related to weight loss:

- If you are one of those people who tends to eat out a lot, make the conscious decision to spend 45 minutes a week meal planning and 1 hour a week shopping for those meals. This will save time (and money) in the long run.
- If others demand too much of your time, learn to be more assertive. You can't spend your days constantly listening or doing things for other people. Learn to say no and never feel guilty about it.
- Sit down, perhaps with a friend, and brainstorm your schedule and the demands placed on you. Often good friends can spot areas of potential flexibility that you may not have thought of.
- Set aside an hour each day for the different tasks you need to do to help continue your weight-loss programme and see what you can let go. Chances are you will find a few low-priority tasks in your schedule that you can let go.

SECRET 5

DITCH DEAD RELATIONSHIPS

Okay, it's time to get a little controversial but I want you to know that I'm writing this from the heart, knowing that thousands of people out there are fat and struggle to lose weight because they are involved in a relationship that is keeping them that way. I remember with fondness Mary, who came to see me several years ago, 38 kilos (6 stone) overweight and complaining that she was feeling depressed and at the end of her tether. During our sessions, it became clear that Mary was married to a bully and what's more, a complete and utter bore. She explained how he was making her life difficult as she made attempts to change her food intake, join the gym and use the techniques I'd taught her. Eventually, Mary decided enough was enough and asked for a divorce.

Hubby John freaked out when she told him in no uncertain terms that the marriage was over. Not surprisingly he begged her to stay but so much had happened and by this point Mary realised that he was bad news and would never change his bad attitude towards her. She is now a sexy size 10 and happy to be back in the dating game. You see, for Mary life was depressing and she was unhappy, always treading on egg shells, wondering what the husband of 20 years would say or do next. 'Good on you, Mary!' I yelled when we met for coffee recently. She had ditched him, and she had ditched the fat as well.

WHY DEAD RELATIONSHIPS MAKE YOU FAT

There are two main reasons why dead relationships keep people fat. First, they are usually depressing and the only beneficiary is the fridge, which is normally stocked full of food – mostly the unhealthy type, or the secret stash of chocolate. In fact, the food cupboard often ends up becoming your new best friend as your other half continues to irritate the pants off you. If you feel you're in a dead relationship then you may have begun to notice that you eat a lot more due to the unhappiness you feel.

Dead relationships are closely linked to emotional eating and if the relationship isn't repaired or finished, then you will probably get fatter and stay fat. The other reason why this happens is that people in dead relationships often find joy in one thing: food. Because there's no excitement, little harmony and no shared goals the only outlet for celebration is eating. Sadly, although painful, the only way to move forward if the relationship is well and truly dead is to end it and move on!

ASSESSING IF IT'S TRULY DEAD

You may be wondering how you decide if a relationship is truly dead. Of course, it's important to try and work through problems and do your best together to put things right, but if you've already done that and find yourself answering 'yes' to each of the following questions, then it's likely to be over and out for you.

- Has the feeling of closeness gone?
- Is your sex life non-existent?
- Do you find it hard to think of the last time you showed each other some affection?
- Maybe you argue too much, or does he/she irritate you when he/she is around?
- Does he/she frequently moan at you and does that make you feel depressed?
- Does the way he/she eats food irritate you?
- Is he/she failing to support you in your quest to lose weight and eat more healthily?
- Does he/she bore you?
- Does he/she make you unhappy?
- Does he/she disrespect you?
- Do you feel physically or mentally abused?
- Do you like it when you're away from your partner?
- Can you no longer call them a friend?
- Would you like your partner to have a personality transplant?
- Do you find it hard to say 'I love you' and mean it?
- Have you tried to put things right?
- Have you been feeling low in this relationship for more than 18 months?

If the answer to all of the above questions is a resounding YES, then it's likely your relationship is dead. But if you answered NO to some of the questions, of course there's hope and you may benefit from some professional relationship counselling.

MAKEOVER YOUR RELATIONSHIP

If you feel your relationship is worth fighting for and want to put the effort in, there are a number of things you can do. Over the years, I have developed a six-point lifeline plan for couples on the edge. Before working through my plan, however, it's important that the two of you are committed to making the relationship work. Commitment is always needed from both parties because if one of you already wants out, there's little hope of the relationship surviving. There has to be a real buy-in from both of you to get the relationship back on track because if you go into my plan half-heartedly, or simply for the sake of the kids, it just won't work.

1. Lay it on the table

Sit down together and agree that during the conversation you will both have the freedom to speak out and clear the air. Never do this process in conjunction with alcohol or after an argument. The atmosphere must be calm so that you are both open and show respect to one another. During this process there are to be no interruptions and you should both agree that you will be open-minded and flexible enough to acknowledge each other's point of view. Doing this will help you identify the core problems and explore each other's emotional needs. I also suggest you take time out from the conversation, as and when needed, to remain calm and focused on what you are there to do. To lay it on the table together, apply the following structure:

- Each partner in turn shares their concerns, frustrations and emotions while the other keeps quiet.
- Afterwards the other partner responds calmly.
- Both of you agree to identify a solution.

2. Admit what you want

You can incorporate this step with the one above. During this part of the process both of you must discuss what it is you want to happen in the future. It's crucial that you are honest because fooling each other simply makes matters worse. Once again, be open with your feelings. Don't be afraid of rejection in admitting your feelings, even if you fear that they won't be reciprocated. Remember, this is all about being open so that plans can be made for the future. If at this point one of you feels the relationship is over, take time out before coming back, discussing and validating that decision.

3. Build an action plan

Having admitted what you both want, now is the time to start building an action plan to make it happen. Remember, all talk and no action achieves nothing and so together write down the immediate actions you can both buy into. For example, if it's you who does all the cooking, day in, day out, then agree to rotate it. Perhaps you can come to an agreement that your partner will encourage you to eat healthier food and do something social together that will also support your weight loss, such as taking up a sport, walking in the countryside or going Salsa dancing. It can also help to put deadlines in place so you are both focused. If you find that you communicate little, perhaps agree to spend 20 minutes each day talking to each other about your day and maybe looking over your action list together.

4. Agree an 'emergency' plan

Of course, life isn't always as simple as agreeing actions and getting on with it. Emotions may get high, frustrations set in and hostility can occur. Because of this, it's important to agree a plan for when this happens. Maybe agree that if one of you is feeling this way, you will sit down at once and allow space for each other without interrupting so that you can air your views and agree immediate action. If tempers run high during this process, agree to take time out before carrying on. Do your best to stay calm because nothing will be achieved by shouting. A good emergency plan is to go for a walk in the fresh air to discuss things as this gives you time away from the restrictive atmosphere of the house.

5. Take it slowly

As you agree to move forward, allow intimacy to return to the relationship gradually. Forcing sex is a definite no-no! Below are a few suggestions for re-introducing the physical side of your relationship:

• Do something that involves gentle intimacy, such as going out for a walk together, hand in hand, or learning massage.

- Simply lie down with each other on the bed and talk about life! Avoid forcing the chat and instead just let it free flow. As you converse, perhaps hold hands or put an arm around your partner.
- Tell each other that for now the sex doesn't matter and it's not important. This helps to take away any pressure. Remember, the more pressure you put on yourselves the more difficult it will be.
- If you're both adventurous, consider sex toys. There's nothing dirty about them and they can be fun and exciting! Show him/her how you like to use them or allow your partner to operate a toy on you. Say no more!
- Agree to date again! Now this can work really well. For example, arrange a dinner date with your partner and have fun as you relax and enjoy each other's company. Arrange it so that when you return home, you have champagne on ice and take it into the bedroom.

6. Celebrate and monitor

As you move forward together, remember there will be times when you'll have to agree to disagree and although a couple, ultimately you are individuals with your own thoughts and beliefs. Agree between yourselves that being different is exciting and healthy because opposites really do attract and this will make you more interesting to each other. Of course, as your relationship evolves, allow time to celebrate as a couple, too. Never stop having fun with each other or being part of a team. Naturally, at times you will need to be patient but relish the thought that you have someone you love, who at times can also be a pain in the backside! Finally, sit down with each other at regular periods to monitor how your relationship is going. Now you can express and discuss feelings, as well as agree actions for the future together.

BE ASSERTIVE WITH THE DRAINERS

Respected people are assertive people, and as you move forward to lose weight, I want to encourage you to be this way. Being with a partner isn't the only type of relationship to consider; there are friendships – and family relationships, too. While most of your relationships will be positive, there may be some family members and friends who like to pull you down and put obstacles in your path. The most constructive way of dealing with these drainers is to become more assertive. Assertiveness ensures that your needs are respected and met, while at the same time you are able to consider the needs of others.

If you are one of those naturally submissive or passive people then at first you may feel uncomfortable being assertive because you prefer to step away from potential confrontation and feel too anxious to say what you think or to express your needs. You may also have misconceptions about what it really means to be assertive. Those who communicate assertively are not pushy or aggressive; being assertive doesn't mean you have to walk all over others to get what you want. In fact, assertive people are interested in other people's feelings though not at the expense of their own. Assertive communicators do so in a non-threatening manner but one that is direct and warm at the same time. They listen, demonstrate empathy and then state their point of view. And assertive people are willing to change their mind, having listened to the opinions of others.

Applying assertive behaviour

There are many ways to use assertive communication on your journey to a slimmer you. Here are a few examples when you can (and really should) stand up for yourself and say what you think is right for you:

- Eating out, when others insist you try a dish loaded in calories.
- When offered a calorific alcoholic or a non-alcoholic drink.
- Being told by friends or family that you look fine the way you are because they want you to stay the same.
- When your partner tells you that he/she doesn't want you to try new healthy foods, or even encourages you to binge on junk food to help keep you fat because of his/her own insecurities.
- After being informed it won't hurt you to have the weekend off from your weight loss plan.

How to be assertive

Becoming assertive takes time and practice. As you make a conscious effort to be more assertive, it can feel a little risky, especially when conversations don't work out as well as you hoped. Learning to communicate assertively combines three components, namely body language, tone of voice and the words you use. Initially, body language is the most powerful of the three. Researchers claim that 55 per cent of initial communication is via body language, with 38 per cent through tone of voice and just 7 per cent is down to the use of words.

How you sit or stand, the gestures you use and even how you look at someone determines body language. Eye contact is critical as it conveys how you see yourself in relation to the other person. For example, if you tend to look down at the floor, this conveys that you are passive or submitting to the power of the other person. If you are hunched up and look awkward, you suggest the other person is more important than you are. However, if you stand too close to someone and raise your voice they are more likely to consider you an aggressive person. Assertive people stand or sit upright, but in a relaxed way with gentle eye contact and an open expression. They speak in a warm, yet direct manner and the tone is even and well paced as they make their point. As they communicate, they offer empathy to show they appreciate the other person's point of view before using the 'I' statement, showing what they want, believe or expect.

'I' statements can include 'I feel', 'I think' and 'I would like' and show you are taking responsibility for your own feelings rather than blaming someone else. For example, you may say 'Thank you for offering me a piece of birthday cake, it looks really nice. However, I have decided for today, I am not eating sweet food'. This isn't you being rude: you are simply showing that you understand why someone is offering you the birthday cake but you are respecting your own right to refuse to eat it. Let's take another scenario as an example, such as when you are with a partner and they say to you, 'Oh tonight, let's have a curry and a bottle of wine'. You may have decided earlier in the day that you don't want to have that kind of meal and so you should reply assertively with, 'That sounds lovely, but today I've decided I want to have a hot chicken salad instead and stay off the wine.' Don't feel guilty for being assertive! I want you to grant yourself permission to be assertive when necessary and remember this isn't you becoming aggressive. As you can now see, there's a big difference between being an aggressive communicator and an assertive one.

Practice, practice, practice!

Learning to be assertive takes time, so practise as much as you can. You could even practise assertive responses in front of a mirror, or have a friend give you feedback and suggestions. Bouncing off a friend is useful because it's important to think about how the other person may react and how you might cope with this. So, if you are ready to be more assertive, use my step-by-step approach below:

- Start off by understanding your usual style of communication. Are you submissive, aggressive or a mixture of both? Think about what makes you the way you are. Is it a fear of not being liked? Perhaps you feel less important than others. Think about a situation you had recently, such as a so-called friend encouraging you to eat chips or ice cream. How could you have dealt with this differently? What would you have done if you were being assertive?

- Think of opportunities in the future when you can behave more assertively. Begin with something easy and build up to more challenging occasions. For example, you may start by refusing pleasantly when someone offers you a chocolate and build up to requesting advice from a waiter on the healthy options available in the restaurant.

- Decide what you want to say before you say it. Think about using the 'I' statements and try to be as specific as you can. For example, 'I'd like to go for a one-hour walk before we go to the cinema'. Always remember when you speak to another person to allow time for them to listen and respond to you.

- Support what you are saying with the way you say it. Check out your body language and the pace and volume of your voice. If what you are saying is serious, then look like you mean it and *be* serious. Smiling may give the indirect message that you don't really mean it and you're not that confident.

- If the other person doesn't seem to be listening or tries to sidetrack you, stick to your point. Repeat yourself calmly until you feel that you are being heard. In assertiveness, this is known as the 'broken record' technique.

- As you listen to the other person, remember that you can negotiate a compromise. Assertiveness is not always about you winning because assertive people are confident enough to be able to change their minds.

- To improve your level of assertiveness, be consistent and afterwards reflect on your conversations. Think through how well you did and what you might do next time to improve the quality of your assertive communication.

ENDING A 'FAT' RELATIONSHIP

If you feel there's no hope for your relationship and it's a complete waste of time working at it, then there's only one answer and that's to close the door and move on. But it's essential that you're absolutely sure before discussing your feelings with someone with whom you have shared a close relationship. Of course, it's never easy or straightforward saying goodbye to someone you have spent time with and had the chance to share experiences with. A relationship that continuously stresses you out, makes you feel depressed or drives you to consume too much food or alcohol to numb the pain, however, is one that cannot continue. There is never an easy way to end a relationship and always, there will be pain involved. Even if you know it's the right thing to do, breaking up can be a huge deal.

So, if you know there's no point working at the relationship (perhaps you have already followed my relationship survival plan), what do you do next? The first rule of thumb has to be honesty. Explain to your partner why you need to move on and be prepared to answer any questions they may put to you. Be sensitive and allow him/her space as the reality hits home. Choosing the right time is also essential – I have known friends to end their relationships at parties or even on Christmas day! There's never a perfect time to say 'it's over', but do think it over and be sensitive to their feelings rather than acting on impulse.

If you're worried that your partner may become aggressive then consider telling them in a public place such as a restaurant because they will be less likely to explode. You may find it hard to get your message across. Consider writing everything down in a letter in advance and hand it to them after you've explained that the relationship is over. Often this works well with people who are more introverted and reflective in nature. Again, be sensitive and allow them time to digest what you are telling them.

And what do you do if children are involved? Studies have shown that keeping a partnership going for the sake of the kids, especially if it exposes them to conflict and a bad atmosphere in the home, is bad for their psychological health and it's far better to split amicably than to stay together until the bitter end – or at least until the family fly the nest! If you're living together or married, breaking up may mean letting go of certain creature comforts and seeing others' sadness as your split can be difficult for them, too. Be prepared to experience a mix of emotions, including anger, grief and fear. These are perfectly natural, so allow yourself time to work through them. Consider seeking support from a life coach or a specialist counsellor to help you through and try not to rush into a new relationship: the thing you need most will be time.

Painful as it may be to acknowledge your relationship is over, often having done so means you can move forward into a life that brings what you want, including the opportunity to grow, both emotionally and spiritually. Moving on to a life you want, albeit perhaps as a singleton, will help you control your eating as food becomes less important in your life. And remember, if your relationship has been one where you were continuously put down, or one in which you were completely bored, it's important to take comfort in the knowledge that ending it signifies the beginning of something new and more exciting, including a new, slimmer you.

Jane's story

In 2002, Jane contacted me. She was desperate to lose weight, to feel like a woman. Jane was a warm, thoughtful and very attractive woman even though she herself didn't think so. I will never forget the time I looked into her eyes and told her that I would help her become the person she wanted to be as the tears rolled down her cheeks. As she sat looking at me, covering her stomach with her arms, I knew deep down how desperate she was to change and sensed a cry for help.

Normally, I am good at distinguishing between genuine people and those who just want to remain a victim. Looking at Jane, she was evidently the former. As we began to talk, I simply asked her the question, 'What is it you actually want?' This is a question I always use to start off my sessions because all too often people spend time analysing why they are the way they are. It's my view that they want a result and often the journey to the result will excite and inspire them so much that any underlying problems are sorted en route. This was certainly the case with Jane, who went on to explain that she had tried diet after diet only to find she lost a few pounds at best.

For the first couple of sessions, I coached Jane to eat better and I conducted a couple of hypnotherapy sessions to help focus her mind on the end result. During the first two weeks, she lost weight and was overjoyed but it was during the third session that I knew something was still not quite right. As we sat there in the comfort of the warm consulting room, I allowed a few seconds of silence to pass by as I looked into her eyes. As time passed and the silence remained, I decided to share my hunch that there was something not quite right. Again, there was a silence and the seconds passed before her eyes began to well up. I explained to her that if it affected her weight, she must share what she was thinking.

Jane began to open up and explained to me that in her eyes, her husband of 20 years was a trigger for her overeating. She went on to tell me that she really didn't like him, they had separate bedrooms, he bored her and she resented him for bullying her in the early years of their marriage. The relief at sharing this with me was quickly evident and for most of our session she continued to pour out her feelings until I asked the question, 'Do you love him?' She replied straightaway with an emphatic 'NO!' Her answer was one of the most unquestionable responses I had ever heard, so I moved on to ask, 'Do you want to leave him then?' At this point she smiled and yelled, 'YES!' The session continued and she explained how she would like to use the hypnotherapy sessions to help clarify her mind on how to leave the relationship.

Eventually, Jane did file for divorce and to this day she proudly says the process of divorce was one of the most positive experiences she has ever had. Of course, there were the financial challenges to work through, but for her the freedom and new lease of life she experienced were as good as winning first prize in the lottery. Her weight continued to drop off before, during and after the divorce and she has gone down from a size 20 to a size 12.

I frequently catch up with Jane and the radiance on her face melts me every time, thinking about the journey she's been on. Years on, and for Jane, life is now very different: she has a new career and a new and amazing partner. In her words, 'Life can be a whole lot lighter with divorce.'

Adam's story

Several years ago, Adam contacted me, fed up to the back teeth that both he and his wife were fat. They were both keen to lose weight for the sake of their newborn child. Adam was very enthusiastic about losing weight and willing to try anything to get the weight off for good. His wife,

Maria, was also determined to become slimmer and each time I talked to her about it, she would categorically state that from now on, a fat body was to be something of the past. She explained that she had always been overweight but for some reason had not found the motivation to lose the pounds. When Adam first met Maria, he was a normal weight, but married life meant his healthy eating habits had gone out of the window. I met Adam and Maria together and while I could see Adam was keen to move forward, Maria seemed to think I had a magic pill to help her lose weight, or that I could go inside her body and lose the weight for her.

I developed a six-week plan for them both and as we kicked off, both seemed to do well with their weight loss. It was nice and steady for the first three weeks, each losing 1.5kg (3lb). I then decided to call in Maria as I was becoming increasingly concerned that her motivation was slacking and she might be losing her focus. However, Maria's attitude was defensive and obstructive to all the suggestions I offered her. Seeing her alone, and with the opportunity to discuss things honestly, it became obvious that she could simply not be bothered and in fact preferred her former sedentary lifestyle. What I also felt was that she was starting to resent the fact that Adam was losing weight, looking more handsome and getting more attention from the ladies. I discussed this with Maria, who replied frankly, 'Oh, he won't keep it up! He's tried and failed before.' I explained to Maria that this was not an attitude that was likely to spur him on and it could potentially affect their relationship. She acknowledged what I had said and agreed to move forward more positively.

As soon as she left my consulting room, I just knew she was saying all the right things but that she wouldn't put them into action. Adam contacted me later that week, very upset, and explained that Maria was actually sabotaging his weight-loss plan by suggesting they order takeaway food and sit in most nights, watching TV. He was becoming frustrated by her actions and now resented her negative attitude. I agreed to see them together, but Maria refused. Adam agreed to see me anyway, as he wanted to move forward with losing weight (which he did). Indeed, he continued to successfully lose weight, while Maria gave up. The resentment later caused Adam to leave Maria after six years of marriage. Seeing her as having held him back, unwilling to support his cause, he had fallen out of love with his wife. Now divorced, thankfully they remain friends for the sake of their young child. Both have gone on to form new relationships and it doesn't take a genius to work out who is the slimmer couple.

USE THE 80–20 RULE

In this chapter, you will find ideas for meal plans based on my 80–20 rule and I have included a suggested meal plan for 12 weeks. In experiencing the plan for yourself, you will begin to understand how it works and soon be able to adapt it for yourself. The good news is that you can include a bit of what you fancy a few times a week so that eating doesn't have to be boring and restrictive. That's the real beauty of the 80–20 rule! Do remember that you need to combine these plans with daily exercise, though (*see also* Secret 10, pages 183–199).

NUTRITIONISTS CAN BE BAD FOR YOUR HEALTH

Having met many nutritionists over the years, I have found that the majority often confuse people because they give conflicting advice on what they can and cannot eat. They also have a tendency to discuss foods that the majority of people have never even heard of and would find expensive to buy on a weekly basis, let alone get their hands on at the local supermarket! Like me, you probably get frustrated by articles claiming one day a certain food is good for you and then the next day, it's bad for you. These food fads really get on my wick! Thankfully, there are some good nutritionists out there, too.

Take Professor David McCarthy, one of the most respected experts in the UK, who refreshingly explained to me that it was fine to occasionally eat a chocolate bar, a bag of chips, a slice of fudge cake and to drink wine in moderation. Professor McCarthy is one of the most inspiring nutritional experts I have met because like me, he sees the real world and takes a sensible view on what food plans work for people. I recall fondly the day when I offered him some wine gums and he gladly accepted them and then went on to eat a chocolate bar!

However, there are those who are of the view that it just cannot be good to enjoy a portion of chips, a bottle of wine or a piece of cake during the week. I have two words for them: GET REAL! Restricted diets in my view simply won't work long term. You may have tried hundreds of them yourself only to find that after a couple of weeks of denying yourself a little bit of junk food, you have ditched your sensible eating plan. So, breathe a big sigh of relief as I'm about to offer you an alternative to make weight loss a bit easier.

Over the last 12 months, I have worked closely with Alison Carman (MBA, BSc, APHNutr), who is a full-time registered nutritionist with thefoodclinic.org. Together, we have developed numerous meal plans for clients based on good old common sense. In doing so, I have ensured these plans are not restrictive and don't cut out a bit of what you fancy. When developing the ideas, I also wanted to offer you some easy-to-buy-for and easy-to-follow recipes and so, courtesy of Alison, you'll find some mouth-watering recipes outlined below.

BREAKFAST IN A GLASS

Breakfast is a vital meal that should never be skipped, even if you are short on time. Lack of time is a prime excuse for pigging out on junk, so here's the perfect breakfast for when you want to eat well but you're on the run. The preparation time is just 5 minutes for this one-person recipe and I'm sure you may already have the ingredients to hand.

1 banana
Small pot (125g/4oz) low-fat natural yoghurt
150ml/¼ pint orange juice
1 tbsp oats

Place all ingredients in a liquidiser or blender and process until smooth. Transfer to a large glass and enjoy that kick-start we all need in the morning! A slow-burn energy feed and plenty of minerals and vitamins will keep you feeling tip-top.

LOW-CAL COTTAGE PIE

Serves 6

Here is the recipe that will feed six people very nicely. It has some great nutritional and 'filling' elements as the pulses and beans it contains will keep you feeling full and satisfied for longer. The preparation time is just 15 minutes and it takes around 45 minutes to cook up this great dish.

1kg (2lb) potatoes, peeled and halved
1 tbsp rapeseed oil
1 medium onion, chopped
1 garlic clove, crushed
300g (10oz) lean minced beef
2 carrots, peeled and sliced
450ml (¾ pint) lo-salt vegetable stock
410g (14½oz) can kidney beans, drained and rinsed
410g (14½oz) can green lentils, drained and rinsed
3 tbsp skimmed milk
Freshly ground black pepper

1. Preheat the oven to 200°C (400°F) Gas 6.
2. Place the potatoes into a pan of boiling water and simmer until tender, about 20 minutes. Meanwhile, heat the oil in a large saucepan and add the onion and garlic. Fry until golden, turning, for about 3 minutes.
3. Stir in the minced beef and carrots, then cook for a further 2 minutes. Add the stock, kidney beans and lentils. Season and bring to the boil. Cover and reduce the heat to a simmer for 20 minutes.
4. Meanwhile, drain the potato and mash with the skimmed milk; season well. Transfer the beef filling to a large ovenproof dish and top with the potato mash. Smooth and decorate with a fork. Bake for 20–25 minutes until the topping is golden.

MACKEREL PÂTÉ
Serves 6

This pâté makes a great filling for sandwiches, bagels and jacket potatoes, plus it only takes about 10 minutes to prepare. Of course it has some great nutritional input from the oily fish, too!

1 small packet (330g/11oz) smoked mackerel fillets
200g (7oz) low-fat cream cheese
Juice of ½ a lemon
Freshly ground black pepper
Handful of chopped parsley or chives (optional)
Wholemeal toast, to serve

Remove the skin and any small bones from the smoked mackerel. Place the fish in a bowl and mash it up with a fork. Combine with the cream cheese, lemon juice, black pepper and herbs, if using. Serve on wholemeal toast.

PITTA PIZZA
Serves 2

Now there's no need to give up pizza when you're watching your weight! The preparation time for this low-fat version is just 10 minutes and it takes about 10 minutes to cook.

Spray oil
2 large wholemeal round pitta breads
4 tbsp tomato purée
50g (2oz) half-fat mozzarella, grated

Choose two of the following toppings: flaked tuna, wafer-thin ham, sweetcorn, sliced pepper or thinly sliced onion

1. Preheat the oven to 200°C (400°F) Gas 6. Spray the baking sheet with oil, add the pittas and transfer to the oven for 5 minutes.
2. Spread tomato purée evenly over the warmed pitta bases and top with grated mozzarella. Finish with your chosen toppings and bake until the cheese has melted, about 8–10 minutes. Serve warm.

LEMON-ROASTED CHICKEN & POTATOES
Serves 4

Not only delicious but fantastically simple to prepare! All the ingredients go into one large roasting pan to cook in the oven for just an hour. Let the oven do the work in developing the sticky-sweet caramelised flavours. And what's more, it takes just 10 minutes to prepare.

450g (14½oz) new potatoes, halved
2 medium onions, peeled and cut into chunks
8 chicken thighs, skin removed
2 lemons, quartered
Sprigs of thyme or rosemary
Freshly ground black pepper
Spray oil

1. Preheat the oven to 200°C (400°F) Gas 6.
2. Arrange the potatoes and onion in a large roasting pan with the chicken thighs.

3. Add the lemon quarters and herb sprigs, then season with black pepper and spritz with oil.
4. Roast for 1 hour, but give the ingredients a stir halfway through cooking to prevent them sticking to the roasting pan.

SKINNY CHIPS
Serves 4

There's no need to miss out on treats like chips while following the 80–20 rule and here's a delicious recipe that reduces any possible impact on your waistline. For best results, make these oven-baked chips with King Edward or Maris Piper potatoes. They take just 10 minutes to prepare and 20–25 minutes to bake.

4 medium potatoes, peeled and sliced into chunky chips
Spray oil

1. Preheat the oven to 240°C (475°F) Gas 9.
2. Place the chips in boiling water and parboil for 5 minutes, then drain and pat dry on kitchen paper or a tea towel.
3. Arrange on a baking sheet and spritz with a little oil to coat. Bake for 20–25 minutes until crisp and golden.

LIGHT MACARONI CHEESE
Serves 6

A satisfying recipe that uses store cupboard ingredients and you can add fresh spinach as an easy way to increase your vegetable intake. The preparation time is 10–15 minutes and the cooking time is around 15–20 minutes.

450g (14½oz) wholewheat macaroni pasta
2 tbsp rapeseed oil
50g (2oz) plain flour
750ml (1¼ pints) skimmed milk
50g (2oz) half-fat mature Cheddar
1 small bag (100g/3½oz) washed spinach
50g (2oz) wholemeal breadcrumbs

1. Preheat the oven to 190°C (375°F) Gas 5.
2. Meanwhile, cook the macaroni according to the directions on the packet. Drain through a colander, then run under the cold tap and stir to prevent the pasta from sticking together.
3. To make the cheese sauce, heat the oil in a medium pan then add the flour and cook, stirring constantly, for 1 minute over a low heat. Slowly add the milk, stirring to prevent any lumps. Simmer for 3–4 minutes, stirring, until the sauce has thickened. Remove from the heat, stir in the cheese and leave to melt.
4. In a large bowl, combine the cheese sauce and macaroni before stirring in the spinach. Transfer to a large ovenproof dish, top with breadcrumbs and bake for 15–20 minutes until golden.

SKINNY CHILLI
Serves 6

A lighter version of this traditional favourite! Preparation takes just 15 minutes and only 25 minutes cooking time.

Serve with brown basmati rice and a crunchy green salad. What could be simpler?

1 tsp rapeseed oil
1 medium onion, chopped
1 garlic clove, crushed
1 large red pepper, deseeded and finely diced
300g (10oz) lean minced beef
1–2 tsp chilli powder or flakes (whatever you have in your store cupboard)
400ml (14fl oz) lo-salt vegetable stock
400g (13oz) can chopped tomatoes
400g (13oz) can green lentils, drained
400g (13oz) can kidney beans, drained and rinsed
2 tbsp tomato purée
Freshly ground black pepper
Freshly cooked brown basmati rice and a crunchy green salad, to serve

1. Heat the oil in a saucepan, add the onion and garlic and cook for 3 minutes until golden. Stir in the red pepper, mince and chilli; cook until the mince has browned, turning occasionally.
2. Add the stock, tomatoes, lentils, kidney beans and tomato purée. Season with black pepper and bring to the boil. Reduce the heat, cover and simmer for 20 minutes before serving with basmati rice and salad.

LEAN TOAD IN THE HOLE

A classic recipe made with low-fat sausages to reduce the fat and calorie content. It takes just 10 minutes to prepare and around 40 minutes to cook.

75g (3oz) plain flour
1 egg
125ml (4fl oz) skimmed milk
4 low-fat pork sausages

1. Preheat the oven to 220°C (425°F) Gas 7.
2. To make the batter, transfer the flour to a large mixing bowl and with your hands, make a well in the centre. Break the egg into the well and whisk it in, drawing the flour into the centre of the well to combine. Gradually whisk in the milk and leave to stand for 20 minutes.
3. Arrange the sausages in a small roasting pan and bake in the top half of the oven for 20 minutes, turning occasionally. Pour over the prepared batter and continue cooking for 20 minutes until the batter is risen and golden. Serve at once.

PERFECT PEA SOUP
Serves 6

Rich in fibre, vitamin C and iron, peas are a great standby to have in the freezer. This wonderful pea soup takes 10 minutes to prepare and is cooked in just 15–20 minutes. You can freeze any leftovers into single portions.

1tbsp rapeseed oil
1 medium onion, chopped
1 garlic clove, crushed
350g (12oz) frozen peas
1 can haricot beans (400g/13oz), drained and rinsed

800ml (1¼ pints) lo-salt vegetable stock
Freshly ground black pepper

1. Heat the oil in a large saucepan and gently fry the
onion and garlic until softened.
2. Add the peas and beans with the vegetable stock;
season well. Bring to the boil, reduce the heat and
simmer for 15–20 minutes.
3. Allow the mixture to cool slightly, then transfer to a
blender or food processor and blend until smooth.
Check the seasoning and serve in warm bowls.

SPICY TORTILLA WRAPS
Serves 4

Have this meal as a Friday night treat. To reduce the fat
content even more, use turkey mince instead of beef. This
recipe takes around 5 minutes to prepare and 15 minutes
to cook.

Spray oil
400g (13oz) extra-lean minced turkey or minced beef
1 medium onion, chopped
1 red pepper, deseeded and chopped
½ tsp hot chilli powder
295g (10½oz) can condensed tomato soup
4 flour tortilla wraps
25g (1oz) half-fat mature Cheddar, grated
Greek yoghurt (0 per cent fat) and shredded lettuce,
to serve

1. Add a spray of oil to a large saucepan and heat

through. Brown the mince before adding the onion and pepper, then cook for a further 5 minutes.

2. Reduce the heat and stir in the chilli powder, soup and 200ml (7fl oz) water. Simmer for 10 minutes.

3. Divide the spicy beef mixture between tortillas and scatter over the cheese. Finish with a spoonful of Greek yoghurt (0 per cent fat) and a small handful of shredded lettuce. Roll up and serve at once.

TURKEY BURGERS
Makes 8 burgers

Using chicken or turkey mince makes a tasty and low fat alternative to a traditional burger. This recipe can be made in advance or frozen in batches for use at a later date, and it makes a great stand-by supper! The prep time is 10 minutes plus half an hour to chill, and the burgers take around 10 minutes to cook.

1¼kg (2.8lbs) lean turkey or chicken mince
1 medium onion, finely chopped
140g (5oz) breadcrumbs
1 egg, beaten
A little salt and freshly ground black pepper
Burger buns
Lettuce leaves and sliced red onion

1. Place the ingredients into a large mixing bowl, season and mix together thoroughly.

2. Divide the mixture into 4 and roll into balls then flatten to make burgers and chill for 30 minutes.

3. Grill burgers under a preheated hot grill, turning once.

Make sure they are thoroughly cooked through before serving in warmed burger buns with lettuce and sliced red onion.

VEGETABLE FRITTATA
Serves 4

The Prep time for this is 10 minutes and takes around 20 minutes to cook.

5ml (1tsp) or a spray of oil
1 large onion, chopped
2 cloves garlic, crushed
Pinch of mild chilli powder
200g (7oz) frozen mixed vegetables (sweet corn/peas/carrots)
4 medium eggs, beaten
Salt and ground black pepper
25g (1oz) half fat cheddar, grated

1. Heat the oil in a frying pan over a medium heat and add the onion and garlic then fry for a few minutes.
2. Stir in the mixed vegetables, stir well and continue to heat for a further few minutes.
3. Beat the eggs together and season then pour into the pan and allow the eggs to start to set (this should take about 3 – 4 minutes).
4. Scatter over the grated cheese and finish off under a hot grill to brown the top and serve with a crunchy salad.

EATING PATTERNS: SOME BASIC PRINCIPLES
It's great to have some delicious recipes to hand that you

know how to shop for and prepare and now we've gone through some of my personal favourites. However, it's essential that you get a handle on your own eating patterns, too. Let me help you to work out your own eating pattern so you know what's right for you. While I don't want to impose restriction, I do want to direct you towards some healthy principles. Follow these guidelines and you won't go wrong:

- Make sure you eat three meals a day, with snacks twice daily.
- Keep your mind occupied between meals so you don't pick at food.
- Stay hydrated: make water your drink of choice. Make sure you drink 6–8 glasses of water each day and reduce your intake of fizzy drinks.
- There is no need to bin fizzy drinks completely. Try having just one a day if you are used to drinking lots of fizzy drinks.
- Enjoy at least five portions of fruit and vegetables a day. Remember, one glass of juice can count as one of your '5 a day' so it's not that difficult.
- Buy pure juice where possible and not those made from concentrates or juice drinks.
- Keep your alcohol intake within recommended weekly safe drinking limits.
- As much as possible cut out the saturated fat found in pies, pasties, pastries, cakes and biscuits, but keep the 80–20 rule in mind: the odd treat is fine.
- Manage your portions by using smaller plates, only cooking small portions and using a portion plate (see page 85), if it helps.
- Get active and build exercise into your daily

routine (check first with your GP what level of exercise is right for you).

- Identify the foods you cannot live without and enjoy 'a little of what you fancy'– occasionally! Remember, portion control is the key.

FOOD DIARY

You may want to consider using a food diary to help remind you of what you are trying to achieve. It's important to know what you are feeding your body and how often; a food diary can help you to do just that. It enables you to monitor and track your progress and many of my clients have benefited. Include the amount of water you drink, frequency of meals and details of your exercise plan. This allows you to accurately track the healthy foods you are enjoying and take note of the treats you are consuming, so you can get the balance right, reinforcing in your own mind the 80–20 rule.

As part of the food diary and recording process, you may want to take a full-length photo of yourself and date it on the back. Include measurements taken from your neck, chest (bust), biceps, waist, hips, thigh and calf and then in three months' time repeat this and compare. This will help you see your progress and acts as another motivational tool.

WHY I LIKE '5 A DAY'

When I was fat, it was rare that I ate a single portion of fruit or vegetables each day, let alone five! When I finally realised that I should be eating '5 a day' to be healthier, I saw this as one huge chore! Over time, however, I started to make this a natural habit and I'm so glad I welcomed it into my life. At first, I thought it would be hard work – how on earth was I going to eat five portions of fruit and vegetables a day? After all, I was working long hours five days a week and weekends were taken up with socialising and drinking lots. But enough was enough, and I decided to give it a go. Not only did I begin to feel physically fitter but my mental health received a boost, too: my concentration improved and I didn't feel quite so mentally drained when I got home from work.

It's true that fruit and vegetables are an important source of nutrition. And, let's face it, you probably already know this but what you're not necessarily doing at the moment is making them part of your daily habit. But before I help you change your eating habits, let's take a look at why it's important to get your five portions:

- Fruit and vegetables taste great and they are important sources of vitamins and minerals, such as vitamin C and potassium, which you need to help maintain a healthy body.
- They are also filled with fibre: this helps maintain a healthy gut and if you suffer from constipation, you will certainly find going to the loo a little more comfortable. And remember, a high-fibre diet reduces the risk of bowel cancer.
- Your '5 a day' will reduce the risk of heart disease and stroke and because fruit and vegetables are low in fat and calories, they will help slim you down, too. That said: if you fry them in oil, the fat increases so be aware of how you cook them!

To help you enjoy eating your '5 a day', do try to use a wide variety of fruit and vegetables. First, this will prevent you from getting bored and second, different fruit and vegetables contain different combinations of fibre, vitamins, minerals and other nutrients. Do remember potatoes do not count towards your '5 a day', though, so no popping them into the count! If you're anything like I was, you are probably wondering what constitutes a portion. Here are a few examples to help you:

- One apple.
- One banana.
- One pear.
- One orange.
- Two plums.
- Two satsumas.
- Half an avocado.
- A large slice of melon or pineapple.
- Cup of grapes or cherries.
- One dessert bowl of salad.
- Small glass of pure fruit or vegetable juice (non-concentrate).
- Two pieces of broccoli or four heaped dessertspoons kale, spinach or spring greens.
- Three heaped tablespoons cooked vegetables, e.g. carrots, peas, sweetcorn, cauliflower.
- Three heaped tablespoons baked beans, kidney beans or chickpeas.

Remember, fruit juice can only count as one portion, no matter how much you drink. But, if you love smoothies (which contain a tasty mix of fruit and/or vegetables) then one of these may also count towards your '5 a day', and the good news is that it may even count towards more than one of your '5 a day'. However, no matter how many you drink, smoothies can only count as a maximum of two of your '5 a day'. Beans and pulses also count as one portion, no matter how much you eat.

PORTION CONTROL

It's not just *what* you put it in; crucially, it's also *how much*! While the 80–20 rule helps keep your food choices realistic, it's no good eating too much of it. You can eat all the right foods in the world but if you intake too many calories and fail to burn them off, you will stay fat or indeed, get fatter. Yes, it's all about quantity as much as quality but what I don't want to do is confuse you by recommending you start to weigh your foods and work through a number of complex calculations that will only make losing weight a real bore and not a pleasure at all. Portion control is, to a large degree, common sense. Here are some examples:

- Four roast potatoes *or* eight roast potatoes?
- Four chunks of chocolate *or* six chunks of chocolate?
- One Yorkshire pudding *or* two?
- One takeaway per week *or* three?
- One banana *or* three?
- Six low-calorie chocolate digestives *or* two?

With portion control, the secret lies in being realistic and sensible – and having a number of tools to train your brain to eat the right amount of food for the long haul, so read on!

Make food invisible

This isn't an abracadabra trick. What I mean is, keep food out of sight so the temptation to nibble is limited.

Share and share alike

When you go out to eat, try sharing side portions with friends and family. Also, only take so much cash out with you and leave your cards at home. I used to do this all the time when eating out; it stopped me from having extra servings and always prevented me drinking too much alcohol.

Slow down

When eating a meal make it last 20 minutes: it takes that amount of time for your hunger to be satisfied. Try sipping water or pure fruit juice as you eat. Be conscious of chewing and tasting your food rather than racing ahead.

Use a portion plate

Portion plates can work really, really well if you are unsure of how much to pop onto your plate. These can be purchased via the Internet. Simply search online 'portion control plates' and you will find a number of options available.

Start leaving food on your plate

As you eat more slowly and your hunger becomes satisfied more easily, do try to leave a little food on your plate. To avoid food waste, store it in a plastic container for another day but if that's not possible, don't feel guilty about throwing it away.

Try meat as a side dish

Something I do every Sunday is make meat a side dish. In doing so, I load my plate full of healthy vegetables, which really fill me up so I eat a very small portion of meat on the side.

Look at your fat photo

If you feel your portions are out of control, consider placing a photo of yourself (one that you despise) close by as you eat your meal. This will make you think twice before going back for seconds!

Implement the fat break

One technique that works very well for my clients is piling food so high on a huge plate that there's far too much to eat. Look at the food, decide how much you're going to eat and simply draw a line on the plate. Eat slowly towards your line and once you have reached it, stop eating. I call this the 'fat break' – you stop at the fat break and put the remainder of your food in a plastic container for another day. Clients often report that this helps affirm that they are in control of food and the food is no longer controlling them.

THE 12-WEEK PLAN

What follows is a sample 12-week meal plan utilising the 80–20 rule, which has been developed by Alison Carman, consultant nutritionist, and myself. The meals are, of course, fabulous for one but it goes without saying that they are great meals which can be made for all the family, as well as visiting friends. Feel free to mix and match as well but make sure you stick to smaller portions!

The 12-week plan

12 WEEK PLAN	BREAKFAST	LUNCH	DINNER	SNACK ON...	A LITTLE OF WHAT YOU FANCY
Day 1: Monday	Enjoy a Lean Bacon Butty! Grill two slices of bacon (fat removed) and serve between two slices of wholemeal bread spread with a little ketchup or brown sauce, plus a glass of juice.	Toss together a small drained can of salmon flakes with half a diced pepper and a handful of cherry tomatoes. Serve with 1 tbsp low-fat mayo on salad leaves.	Grilled chicken breast (skin removed) served with potatoes, broccoli and carrots, plus a glass of orange juice.	A crunchy apple or a nice cuppa with semi-skimmed milk and a plain biscuit.	
Day 2: Tuesday	A hearty bowl of chopped fresh fruit served with a small pot of low-fat yoghurt.	A serving of Perfect Pea Soup (see page xx) with two wholemeal crackers (reserve the other portion for Thursday).	Grill two lean lamb chops. Serve with a small baked potato and freshly cooked green beans.	Small handful of salted popcorn or a banana.	

12 WEEK PLAN	BREAKFAST	LUNCH	DINNER	SNACK ON...	A LITTLE OF WHAT YOU FANCY
Day 3: Wednesday	25g (1oz) muesli served with semi-skimmed milk and a handful of raspberries, plus a small glass of your favourite juice.	Egg mayo (low-fat) on two thick slices of granary bread.	Throw together a simple tuna salad. In a bowl, toss 1 tbsp of low-fat dressing with a small can of drained tuna flakes, a handful of boiled new potatoes, salad leaves and a chopped spring onion.	A handful of grapes or a small skinny latte.	Packet of baked or 'Lite' crisps to enjoy with your sandwich at lunch.
Day 4: Thursday	A couple of slices of thick granary toast spread with low-fat cream cheese and one apple or pear.	Heat the remaining vegetable soup from Tuesday and serve with two crackers and a piece of fruit.	Tuck into Lean Spaghetti Bolognese made with lean beef mince, no added oil and a small low-fat jar of Bolognese sauce. Serve with 6 tbsp cooked wholemeal pasta and a portion of mixed vegetables.	Low-fat cottage cheese spread over two oatcakes and an orange.	Two delicious scoops low-fat ice cream.

12 WEEK PLAN	BREAKFAST	LUNCH	DINNER	SNACK ON...	A LITTLE OF WHAT YOU FANCY
Day 5: Friday	25g (1oz) porridge oats made with semi-skimmed milk served with chunks of banana, plus a nice cuppa made with semi-skimmed milk.	Grab a low-fat ready made chicken salad from your local store.	Grill a piece of fish (choose from cod, haddock or any other firm white fish). Serve with a crunchy salad and 5–6 small new potatoes.	An apple.	Enjoy your favourite tipple – this may be a glass of red or white wine, a beer or spirit with a slim-line mixer.
Day 6: Saturday	Breakfast in a Glass (see page 69).	A portion of Mackerel Pâté (see page 71) served on a slice of wholemeal toast with cucumber and tomato slices.	Fish and chips from the local chippy – choose the small portion and share the chips with a friend!	Veggie sticks – try carrot and celery.	

12 WEEK PLAN	BREAKFAST	LUNCH	DINNER	SNACK ON...	A LITTLE OF WHAT YOU FANCY
Day 7: Sunday	Sliced grilled mushrooms on wholemeal toast.	Tuck into a Lean Roast Dinner but limit your roast spuds to three to four small ones and fill up on three choices of vegetable.	Throw together a Veggie Stir-Fry using half a bag of stir-fry vegetables, 1 tbsp rapeseed oil and a small portion of noodles. Flavour the veggies with 1 tbsp Chinese five spice while cooking.	Two pieces of your favourite fruit.	A glass of your favourite tipple.
Day 8: Monday	Two slices wholemeal toast with low-sugar jam or marmalade, plus a glass of orange juice.	One portion of mixed bean or lentil soup with a wholemeal roll.	Lean grilled gammon steak with 3 tbsp mixed veggies and a portion of Skinny Chips (see page 73).	A piece of fruit or a small handful of almonds.	
Day 9: Tuesday	McDonald's Double Bacon & Egg McMuffin.	Wholemeal pitta filled with tuna and low-fat mayo mixed with diced cucumber and pepper.	6 tbsp cooked wholemeal pasta served with readymade tomato sauce and 3 tbsp mixed vegetables.	A small skinny latte or a nice cuppa and a plain biscuit or an orange.	

90

12 WEEK PLAN	BREAKFAST	LUNCH	DINNER	SNACK ON...	A LITTLE OF WHAT YOU FANCY
Day 10: Wednesday	One chocolate Weetabix with semi-skimmed milk and a chunk of sliced banana.	Chicken Salad (salad leaves, tomatoes and cucumber) with low-fat Caesar dressing Go easy on the Parmesan.	Two egg mushroom omelette with half-fat Cheddar served with a large green salad.	An apple.	One small piece chocolate cake.
DAY 11: Thursday	Chunks of fruit (try pineapple and melon) with low-fat yoghurt.	Toasted Croque Monsieur made with half-fat Cheddar and lean ham between two slices wholemeal bread.	Jacket potato with prawns in low-fat cocktail sauce, plus a huge bowl of crunchy mixed salad.	Carrot sticks and low-fat dip or a banana.	

12 WEEK PLAN	BREAKFAST	LUNCH	DINNER	SNACK ON...	A LITTLE OF WHAT YOU FANCY
Day 12: Friday	Dip chunky wedges of wholemeal toast soldiers (two slices) into two medium sized soft-boiled eggs.	Leftover vegetable soup! Chop up any veggies left over in your fridge, such as carrots, peppers or beans and an onion. Heat a pint of vegetable stock and add your chopped vegetables. Leave to simmer for 25 minutes, then whizz in a blender until smooth. Reheat and serve a portion with a wholemeal roll.	Lean grilled beefsteak served with potato wedges. Cut one medium potato into chunks and place on a baking sheet, spray with a little oil and bake in a hot oven (180°C/350°F/Gas 4) for 20–25 minutes. Serve with green beans or peas.	Two oatcakes.	A glass of your favourite tipple.
Day 13: Saturday	25g (1oz) muesli with semi-skimmed milk and grapes, plus a glass of juice.	Shop-bought low-calorie chicken Caesar wrap or sandwich.	Your favourite take-away (e.g. KFC, McDonald's or Pizza Hut, but watch the portion size!).	Two pieces of fruit.	

12 WEEK PLAN	BREAKFAST	LUNCH	DINNER	SNACK ON...	A LITTLE OF WHAT YOU FANCY
Day 14: Sunday	Low-fat yoghurt and a piece of fruit.	Light Macaroni Cheese (see page 73) with a handful of lean diced ham and a side of mixed salad.	Sardines on a thick slice of wholemeal toast with a few cherry tomatoes.	An apple.	A glass of your favourite tipple.
Day 15: Monday	Whizz up scrambled eggs on a toasted crumpet. Serve with a glass of juice.	Grab a low-cal sandwich to go and a ready prepared fruit salad.	Grilled fresh tuna steak with a huge bowl of mixed salad.	An apple.	Indulge in a low-calorie hot chocolate and a plain biscuit.
Day 16: Tuesday	Grilled tomatoes on wholemeal bread.	Half a carton or half a can of chunky vegetable soup with a wholemeal roll.	Grilled chicken breast (skin removed) served with potatoes, broccoli and carrots.	A small skimmed milk latte or an apple.	
Day 17: Wednesday	25g (1oz) porridge oats or a ready measured sachet made with semi-skimmed milk, plus an apple.	Wholemeal pasta mixed with chopped peppers and cucumber, flaked canned salmon and 1 tbsp low-fat dressing.	A portion of Vegetable Frittata (see page 79), served with a mixed salad.	Fun-size packet dried raisins or apricots; carrot sticks.	

12 WEEK PLAN	BREAKFAST	LUNCH	DINNER	SNACK ON...	A LITTLE OF WHAT YOU FANCY
Day 18: Thursday	One chocolate Weetabix with semi-skimmed milk and a handful of raspberries.	Mixed Bean Salad. To make this, drain and rinse a small can of mixed beans. Place in a bowl and stir in 3 tbsp defrosted mixed vegetables. Crumble over 25g (1oz) feta cheese. Serve with 1 tbsp low-fat dressing.	Oven-Baked Chicken. Preheat the oven to 200°C (400°F) Gas 6. Place a chicken breast (skin removed) in a foil package with a little chicken stock and 1 tbsp white wine. Bake for 25 minutes and serve with two types of vegetable.	Two pieces of fruit.	A glass of your favourite tipple.
Day 19: Friday	McDonald's Low Fat Blueberry Muffin with a large regular black or white coffee.	Homemade or shop-bought leek & potato soup with a granary roll.	Turkey Burger (see page 78) in a bun and homemade Skinny Chips (page 73) with a large green salad.	A handful of grapes or an apple.	
Day 20: Saturday	Try our skinny grilled English breakfast: Tuck	Wholemeal pitta filled with tuna and low-fat	A portion of Lean Toad in the Hole (see page 75)	One banana.	Two scoops of sorbet.

12 WEEK PLAN	BREAKFAST	LUNCH	DINNER	SNACK ON...	A LITTLE OF WHAT YOU FANCY
	into two grilled slices of back bacon, grilled mushrooms and tomatoes (spray with a little oil) and serve with low-sugar baked beans.	mayo mixed with diced cucumber or pepper.	served with freshly cooked carrots and peas.		
Day 21: Sunday	Enjoy a large bowl of fruit salad – try a combination of melon, apple and mango.	Tuck into a Lean Roast Dinner (see page 90).	Throw together a Veggie Stir-Fry (see page 90).	An orange and a small bunch of grapes.	A glass of your favourite tipple.
Day 22: Monday	A hearty bowl of fruit salad and a small pot of yoghurt.	Jacket potato with low-sugar baked beans.	Enjoy a ready prepared vegetable lasagne.	One banana.	One low-sugar fruit jelly.

12 WEEK PLAN	BREAKFAST	LUNCH	DINNER	SNACK ON...	A LITTLE OF WHAT YOU FANCY
Day 23: Tuesday	25g (1oz) porridge oats or a ready measured sachet made with semi-skimmed milk and served with chunks of banana; a nice cuppa with semi-skimmed milk.	Create a Salade Niçoise. Slice a tomato and a 10cm (4in) piece of cucumber into chunks. Place in a bowl and toss in half a finely chopped red onion, a small can of tuna (drained), anchovies and olives. Drizzle with 1 tbsp low-fat dressing and top with soft-boiled egg slices.	Grilled salmon fillet served with roasted vegetables. To make the vegetables, preheat the oven to 200°C (400°F) Gas 6. Meanwhile, deseed and cut a pepper into chunks along with one courgette and a small onion. Spray with a little oil, season and roast for 20 minutes.	Two oatcakes or a plain biscuit and a nice cuppa.	
Day 24: Wednesday	25g (1oz) muesli with semi-skimmed milk and grapes.	Half a carton or can of vegetable soup with a wholemeal roll.	Two-egg omelette with a little grated half-fat Cheddar and a large mixed salad.	Fun-size pack of raisins or one apple.	
Day 25: Thursday	Toasted bagel with low-sugar jam; one banana.	Enjoy a smoked salmon sandwich with lettuce	6 tbsp cooked wholemeal pasta served with ready	An apple.	Indulge in a small bag of your

12 WEEK PLAN	BREAKFAST	LUNCH	DINNER	SNACK ON...	A LITTLE OF WHAT YOU FANCY
		between two slices of wholemeal bread.	made vegetable sauce.		favourite crisps.
Day 26: Friday	Stew some plums, rhubarb or apple and serve with a small pot of low-fat yoghurt. Sprinkle 1 tbsp muesli over the top.	Pasta salad made with wholemeal cooked pasta, one slice of ham (cut into strips), chopped peppers and cucumber, plus 1 tbsp low-fat dressing. Perfect for your lunch box!	Grilled Chicken Breast (skin removed) with Egg-Fried Rice. Heat a spray of oil in a wok, then stir-fry two chopped spring onions and half a diced pepper. Add a cup of cooked rice. Crack in two medium sized eggs and stir to allow the eggs to scramble.	A banana or carrot sticks.	A glass of your favourite tipple.
Day 27: Saturday	Lean Bacon Butty (see page 87), plus a glass of juice.	Small tub hummus served with a selection of crunchy vegetable sticks, such as celery, carrot, pepper and cucumber.	Light Macaroni Cheese (see page 73) with a mixed salad.	Handful of berries or three breadsticks.	

12 WEEK PLAN	BREAKFAST	LUNCH	DINNER	SNACK ON...	A LITTLE OF WHAT YOU FANCY
Day 28: Sunday	Grilled mushrooms or tomatoes on wholemeal toast, plus a glass of orange juice.	A portion of Low-Cal Cottage Pie (see page 69) with two choices of vegetable.	In a large bowl, toss together a small can of salmon (drained and flaked with a fork), half a pepper (deseeded and diced) and a handful of cherry tomatoes. Serve on salad leaves.	Two pieces of fruit.	Enjoy a glass of your favourite tipple.
Day 29: Monday	Stew some cooking apples and serve with a small pot of yoghurt, sprinkled with 1 tbsp muesli plus a glass of orange juice.	A portion of Mackerel Pâté (see page 71) served on wholemeal toast.	Make your favourite Spaghetti Bolognese recipe using turkey mince (see page 88). Serve with wholemeal pasta and broccoli.	A banana or carrot sticks.	
Day 30: Tuesday	A small bowl of Bran Flakes or one Weetabix served with a handful of strawberries and semi-	Treat yourself to a low-fat chicken and salad sandwich from your local supermarket plus a small	Grilled pork chop (fat removed) with a large helping of ratatouille.	Two oatcakes or an apple.	One small piece of chocolate cake or a small chocolate bar (25g/1oz).

12 WEEK PLAN	BREAKFAST	LUNCH	DINNER	SNACK ON...	A LITTLE OF WHAT YOU FANCY
	skimmed milk.	pot of low-calorie fruit yoghurt.			
Day 31: Wednesday	Scrambled eggs on wholemeal toast.	Jacket potato with low-sugar baked beans.	Put together a Veggie and Cashew Nut Stir-Fry using half a bag of prepared stir-fry vegetables and a small portion of noodles. Add a small handful of cashews just before serving.	An orange or a small bunch of grapes.	
Day 32: Thursday	A great standby − two pancakes made with semi-skimmed milk and served with defrosted frozen mixed berries.	Wholemeal pitta filled with tuna and low-fat mayo mixed with diced cucumber or pepper.	Light Macaroni Cheese (see page 73) served with a choice of two veggies.	Nice cuppa with a reduced fat digestive; an apple.	

12 WEEK PLAN	BREAKFAST	LUNCH	DINNER	SNACK ON...	A LITTLE OF WHAT YOU FANCY
Day 33: Friday	Lean Bacon Butty (see page 87) and a glass of orange juice.	Half a carton or half a can of chunky vegetable soup with a wholemeal roll.	Large takeaway Thin & Crispy Vegetable & Ham Pizza.	A banana or vegetables sticks, such as cucumber or pepper.	A glass of your favourite tipple.
Day 34: Saturday	Tuck into a bowl of chopped apple and pineapple served with a dollop of Greek yoghurt (0 per cent fat).	Croque Monsieur (see page 91).	Serve a steaming bowl of freshly cooked tagliatelle with 125g (4oz) mixed seafood sautéed in a spritz of oil and crushed garlic.	An apple.	Low-fat chocolate mousse for dessert.
Day 35: Sunday	Toasted bagel with low-sugar marmalade, plus one apple.	Tuck into a Lean Roast Dinner (see page 90).	Egg mayo sandwich with shredded green lettuce between two slices of wholemeal bread.	Fun-size pack of dried fruit; three breadsticks.	Enjoy a glass of your favourite tipple.
Day 36: Monday	25g (1oz) muesli with semi-skimmed milk and	Leftover vegetable soup (see page 92).	Grilled fresh tuna steak with a huge bowl of mixed	A nice cuppa made with semi-skimmed	

12 WEEK PLAN	BREAKFAST	LUNCH	DINNER	SNACK ON...	A LITTLE OF WHAT YOU FANCY
	chunks of apple.		salad; bowl of strawberries.	milk and a plain biscuit or an apple.	
Day 37: Tuesday	Two toasted crumpets with low-sugar jam or marmalade and a glass of orange juice.	Grab a ready prepared pasta salad but make sure it contains at least one of your five-a day!	Two-egg omelette with one slice of lean ham (diced) and a large mixed salad.	One banana.	A bar of milk chocolate (25g/1oz).
Day 38: Wednesday	Dip chunky wedges of wholemeal toast soldiers (two slices) into two medium sized soft-boiled eggs. Serve with a glass of your favourite juice.	Jacket potato with cottage cheese and pineapple.	6 tbsp cooked wholemeal pasta served with ready made tomato sauce and 3 tbsp mixed vegetables.	Two oatcakes or a piece of fruit.	

12 WEEK PLAN	BREAKFAST	LUNCH	DINNER	SNACK ON...	A LITTLE OF WHAT YOU FANCY
Day 39: Thursday	Low-sugar baked beans on wholemeal toast.	Tuna Wrap. Simply spread a wrap with 1 tbsp low-fat mayo. Top with shredded lettuce, cucumber and tomato slices and 2 tbsp flaked tuna. Tuck in the ends, roll up and enjoy!	Grilled chicken breast (skin removed) served with potatoes, broccoli and carrots.	Fun-size packet dried fruit or carrot sticks.	
Day 40: Friday	Two stewed peaches served with a dollop of Greek yoghurt (0 per cent fat).	Mackerel Pâté (see page 71) served on a slice of thick wholemeal toast and with a handful of sliced cherry tomatoes on the side.	A portion of Lean Toad in the Hole (see page 75) serve with freshly cooked carrots and green beans.	One orange.	Two Jaffa Cakes or a glass of your favourite tipple.
Day 41: Saturday	McDonald's Big Breakfast, an apple.	Half a can of lentil soup served with a wholemeal bread roll.	A portion of Spicy Tortilla Wraps (see page 77).	Small bunch of grapes.	

12 WEEK PLAN	BREAKFAST	LUNCH	DINNER	SNACK ON...	A LITTLE OF WHAT YOU FANCY
Day 42: Sunday	25g (1oz) muesli with semi-skimmed milk and chunks of banana.	Tuck into a Lean Roast Dinner (see page 90).	Sardines on a thick slice of wholemeal toast with cucumber slices.	Two pieces of fruit.	A glass of your favourite tipple.
Day 43: Monday	Lean Bacon Butty (see page 87).	A serving of Perfect Pea Soup (see page 76) with two wholemeal crackers.	Preheat the oven to 190°C (375°F) Gas 5. Remove the skin from a chicken breast, spread with 1 tbsp pesto and bake for 20 minutes. Serve with a large mixed salad.	Two crabsticks or a banana.	
Day 44: Tuesday	Breakfast in a Glass (see page 69). This time vary the recipe by adding a handful of berries.	Half an avocado (sliced) served with a handful of cooked prawns and shredded lettuce. Finish with 1 tbsp low-calorie Thousand Island dressing.	A portion of Low-Cal Cottage Pie (see page 69). Serve with two choices of vegetable.	A crunchy apple or a nice cuppa with semi-skimmed milk and a plain biscuit.	

103

12 WEEK PLAN	BREAKFAST	LUNCH	DINNER	SNACK ON...	A LITTLE OF WHAT YOU FANCY
Day 45: Wednesday	Whizz up scrambled eggs on a toasted crumpet. Serve with a glass of juice.	Small tub hummus served with a selection of crunchy vegetable sticks, such as celery, carrot, pepper and cucumber.	Sliced Beef & Beetroot Salad. Place a handful of shredded lettuce in a pasta bowl. Top with two slices lean beef, beetroot and cucumber slices, finished off with a dollop of Greek yoghurt (0 per cent fat).	Three breadsticks.	Low-sugar jelly.
Day 46: Thursday	25g (1oz) muesli served with semi-skimmed milk and a handful of raspberries, plus a glass of your favourite juice.	Mixed Bean Salad. Drain and rinse a small can of mixed beans. Transfer to a large bowl and stir in 3 tbsp defrosted mixed vegetables. Crumble 25g (1oz) feta cheese over the top and serve with 1 tbsp low-fat dressing.	Tuck into a Lean Spaghetti Bolognese (see page 88). Serve with 6 tbsp cooked wholemeal pasta and a portion of mixed vegetables.	A small skinny latte.	A chocolate biscuit.

12 WEEK PLAN	BREAKFAST	LUNCH	DINNER	SNACK ON...	A LITTLE OF WHAT YOU FANCY
Day 47: Friday	Chopped apple and banana with a small low-fat fruit yoghurt.	Low-Fat Egg Mayo Salad. Chop up a hardboiled egg and mix with 1 tbsp low-calorie mayo. Serve with a crunchy salad.	Spoil yourself with a Fish Finger Samie! Bake two fish fingers and serve in a wholemeal roll with sliced gherkins and a side of Skinny Chips (see page 73).	Two pieces of fruit.	A glass of your favourite tipple.
Day 48: Saturday	A small bowl of Bran Flakes or one Weetabix served with a handful of strawberries and semi-skimmed milk.	Two slices lean pork in a toasted wholemeal pitta with 1 tbsp low-calorie coleslaw.	Two-egg mushroom omelette with diced lean ham. Serve with a large green salad.	Handful of grapes.	
Day 49: Sunday	Grilled mushrooms or tomatoes on wholemeal toast.	A portion of Lean Toad in the Hole (see page 75), served with freshly cooked carrots and peas.	In a large bowl, toss together a small can of salmon flakes (drained) with half a pepper (deseeded and diced) and a handful of cherry tomatoes. Serve on salad leaves.	Carrot or cucumber sticks.	A glass of your favourite tipple.

12 WEEK PLAN	BREAKFAST	LUNCH	DINNER	SNACK ON...	A LITTLE OF WHAT YOU FANCY
Day 50: Monday	Two slices wholemeal toast spread thinly with Marmite and one crunchy apple.	Greek Salad. Arrange chopped tomatoes and cucumber over shredded lettuce with 4–5 black olives and sprinkle with 1 tbsp crumbled feta.	Lean grilled gammon steak with 3 tbsp mixed veggies or a large mixed salad.	A nice cuppa with semi-skimmed milk and a plain biscuit.	
Day 51: Tuesday	Low-sugar baked beans on wholemeal toast and a glass of orange juice.	Egg mayo (low-fat) on two thick slices of granary bread with a handful of halved cherry tomatoes.	Tuna & Potato Salad. In a bowl, combine six halved new potatoes with chopped cucumber and two diced spring onions. Add half a can of drained, flaked tuna and one tablespoon of low calorie mayo. Toss together.	Low-fat cottage cheese spread over two oatcakes.	A bar of chocolate (25g/1oz).
Day 52: Wednesday	A hearty bowl of fruit salad and a small pot of yoghurt.	Mug of instant vegetable soup with two oatcakes; one banana.	6 tbsp cooked wholemeal pasta served with ready made vegetable sauce.	Crabsticks or carrot sticks.	

12 WEEK PLAN	BREAKFAST	LUNCH	DINNER	SNACK ON...	A LITTLE OF WHAT YOU FANCY
Day 53: Thursday	A toasted crumpet topped with slices of strawberry and a teaspoon of runny honey.	One large slice of rye bread spread with low-fat cottage cheese and pineapple.	Roasted chicken breast (skin removed) spread with 1 tbsp sun-dried tomato paste and baked in a hot oven (190°C/375°F/Gas 5) for 20 minutes. Serve with a large mixed salad.	Fun-size packet dried raisins or apricots.	
Day 54: Friday	McDonald's Big Breakfast.	Shop-bought low-calorie Chicken Caesar wrap or sandwich.	A portion of Spicy Tortilla Wraps (see page 77).	Two small Clementines.	A glass of your favourite tipple.
Day 55: Saturday	Half a ruby grapefruit and a small pot of low-fat yoghurt.	Enjoy a Skinny Brunch! Tuck into two grilled slices of back bacon, grilled mushrooms and tomatoes (spray with a little oil) and serve with low-sugar baked beans.	Grill a piece of fish (choose from cod, haddock or any other firm white fish). Serve with a crunchy salad and five to six small new potatoes.	One apple.	Individual low-calorie trifle or chocolate mousse.

12 WEEK PLAN	BREAKFAST	LUNCH	DINNER	SNACK ON...	A LITTLE OF WHAT YOU FANCY
Day 56: Sunday	One Weetabix served with a handful of berries and semi-skimmed milk.	Tricolore Salad. Arrange half a sliced avocado and a large sliced tomato over shredded lettuce leaves. Top with two slices low-fat mozzarella and serve drizzled with 1 tbsp low-calorie Italian dressing.	Treat yourself to Lean Egg & Chips! Cook two medium sized fried eggs in a small spray of oil and serve with our homemade Skinny Chips (see page 73).	One apple or a handful of berries.	A glass of your favourite tipple.
Day 57: Monday	Breakfast in a Glass (see page 69).	Small tub hummus served with a selection of crunchy vegetable sticks, such as celery, carrot, pepper and cucumber.	Portion of Lemon-Roasted Chicken & Potatoes (see page 72), served with broccoli and carrots.	A nice cuppa with semi-skimmed milk and a plain biscuit.	
Day 58: Tuesday	Enjoy a toasted raisin bagel spread with low-sugar jam and a nice cuppa!	Half a can of chunky vegetable soup with a wholemeal roll.	Pitta Pizza (see page 71), served with a mixed salad.	Two pieces of fruit.	

12 WEEK PLAN	BREAKFAST	LUNCH	DINNER	SNACK ON...	A LITTLE OF WHAT YOU FANCY
Day 59: Wednesday	25g (1oz) muesli served with semi-skimmed milk and a handful of raspberries, plus a glass of your favourite juice.	Wholemeal pitta filled with flaked tuna and low-fat mayo mixed with diced cucumber and pepper.	One serving of ready-to-cook mussels served with a portion of French beans and a crusty bread roll.	A small skinny latte.	A chocolate biscuit.
Day 60: Thursday	Chunks of fruit (try pineapple and melon) with low-fat yoghurt.	Jacket potato with low-sugar baked beans.	Veggie Stir-Fry (see page 90).	Fun-size packet dried fruit or carrot sticks.	
Day 61: Friday	One Weetabix served with a sliced banana and semi-skimmed milk.	A portion of Mackerel Pâté (see page 71) served on a thick slice of wholemeal toast with cucumber chunks on the side.	Fish & Chips from your local chippy! Choose a small portion and share the chips with a friend.	An apple or a handful of berries.	

12 WEEK PLAN	BREAKFAST	LUNCH	DINNER	SNACK ON...	A LITTLE OF WHAT YOU FANCY
Day 62: Saturday	Lean Bacon Butty (see page 87).	Grilled Chicken Breast (skin removed) with Egg-Fried Rice. For the rice, heat a spritz of oil and stir-fry a couple of chopped spring onions and half a diced pepper. Stir in a cup of cooked rice. Crack in two medium sized eggs and stir to allow the eggs to scramble. Serve at once.	Tuck into Lean Spaghetti Bolognese (see page 88).	Small bunch of grapes or vegetable sticks.	
Day 63: Sunday	Whizz up scrambled egg on a toasted crumpet and serve with a slice of smoked salmon. Serve with a glass of juice.	Tuck into a Lean Roast Dinner (see page 90).	Half a can of chunky vegetable soup or a serving of Perfect Pea Soup (see page 76) with a wholemeal roll.	Low-fat cottage cheese spread over two oatcakes.	A glass of your favourite tipple.

12 WEEK PLAN	BREAKFAST	LUNCH	DINNER	SNACK ON...	A LITTLE OF WHAT YOU FANCY
Day 64: Monday	25g (1oz) porridge oats or a ready measured sachet made with semi-skimmed milk. Serve with chunks of banana.	Egg mayo (low-fat) on two thick slices of granary bread with a handful of sliced cherry tomatoes.	Homemade Turkey Burger in a bun (see page 78), plus a large green salad.	A nice cuppa with semi-skimmed milk and a plain biscuit.	
Day 65: Tuesday	A hearty bowl of fruit salad and a small pot of yoghurt.	A serving of Perfect Pea Soup (see page 76) with two wholemeal crackers.	A serving of Vegetable Frittata (see page 79), served with a mixed salad.	An orange or a small bunch of grapes.	
Day 66: Wednesday	Dip chunky wedges of wholemeal toast soldiers (two slices) into two medium sized soft-boiled eggs.	Grab a ready prepared pasta salad but make sure it contains at least one of your '5 a day'!	Roasted Chicken Breast with Pesto and a large mixed salad (see page 107).	Crabsticks or an apple.	Small pot of low-fat chocolate mousse.
Day 67: Thursday	Sliced grilled mushrooms on toast.	Enjoy a Salade Niçoise (see page 96).	Grill a piece of fish (cod, haddock or any other firm white fish). Serve with a crunchy salad and five to six small new potatoes.		

12 WEEK PLAN	BREAKFAST	LUNCH	DINNER	SNACK ON...	A LITTLE OF WHAT YOU FANCY
Day 68: Friday	Low-sugar baked beans on wholemeal toast.	One large slice of rye bread spread with low-fat cottage cheese and pineapple.	Your favourite takeaway (KFC, McDonald's or Pizza Hut) – but watch the portion size!	Carrot or cucumber sticks.	Glass of your favourite tipple.
Day 69: Saturday	Chopped apple and banana with a low-fat fruit yoghurt.	A portion of Lean Toad in the Hole (see page 75) with freshly cooked carrots and peas.	Half a can of chunky vegetable soup with a wholemeal roll.	Three breadsticks or a small bunch of grapes.	
Day 70: Sunday	25g (1oz) muesli served with semi-skimmed milk and a handful of berries, plus a glass of your favourite juice.	Skinny Ploughman's. Arrange on a platter one hard-boiled egg (quartered), 40g (1½oz) half-fat Cheddar, one large tomato and a spoonful of Ploughman's pickle. Serve with a crusty roll.	Lemon Roasted Chicken & Potatoes (see page 72) with two choices of vegetable.	Two pieces of fruit.	A glass of your favourite tipple.

12 WEEK PLAN	BREAKFAST	LUNCH	DINNER	SNACK ON...	A LITTLE OF WHAT YOU FANCY
Day 71: Monday	One Weetabix with a handful of strawberries and semi-skimmed milk.	Tuna Wrap. Spread a wrap with 1 tbsp low-fat mayo. Top with shredded lettuce and slices of cucumber and tomato, plus 2 tbsp tuna flakes. Tuck in the ends, roll up and enjoy!	6 tbsp cooked wholemeal pasta served with readymade tomato sauce with a small can of flaked tuna (drained) mixed in.	A nice cuppa with semi-skimmed milk and a plain biscuit.	
Day 72: Tuesday	Poached or scrambled egg on wholemeal toast.	Jacket potato with cottage cheese and pineapple.	6 tbsp cooked wholemeal pasta served with ready made tomato sauce with 3 tbsp mixed vegetables.	Two pieces of fruit.	
Day 73: Wednesday	Breakfast in a Glass (see page 69).	Two slices lean pork in a toasted wholemeal pitta with 1 tbsp low-calorie coleslaw.	Sardines on a thick slice of wholemeal toast with a few sliced cherry tomatoes.	A small skinny latte or an apple.	A chocolate biscuit.

12 WEEK PLAN	BREAKFAST	LUNCH	DINNER	SNACK ON...	A LITTLE OF WHAT YOU FANCY
Day 74: Thursday	Stew some plums, rhubarb or apple in a little sugar and water. Serve with a small pot low-fat yoghurt and 1 tbsp muesli sprinkled over the top.	Small tub hummus served with a selection of crunchy vegetable sticks, such as celery, carrot, pepper and cucumber.	Tuck into Lean Spaghetti Bolognese (see page 88).	Fun-size packet dried fruit or carrot sticks.	
Day 75: Friday	McDonald's Double Bacon & Egg McMuffin.	Chicken salad with low-fat Caesar dressing (include salad leaves, tomato and cucumber slices). Go easy on the Parmesan!	A portion of Low-Cal Cottage Pie (see page 69) with a choice of two vegetables.	Low-fat cottage cheese spread over two oatcakes.	A glass of your favourite tipple or a small slice of chocolate cake.
Day 76: Saturday	Chunks of fruit (try pineapple and melon) with low-fat yoghurt.	Mackerel Pâté (see page 71) on a thick slice of wholemeal toast with a handful of sliced cherry tomatoes.	Enjoy a large takeaway Thin & Crispy Vegetable & Ham Pizza.	Small bunch of grapes or vegetable sticks.	

114

12 WEEK PLAN	BREAKFAST	LUNCH	DINNER	SNACK ON...	A LITTLE OF WHAT YOU FANCY
Day 77: Sunday	A small bowl of Bran Flakes or one Weetabix served with a sliced banana and semi-skimmed milk.	Tuck into a Lean Roast Dinner (see page 90).	Tuna & Potato Salad. In a bowl, combine six halved new potatoes with chopped cucumber and two diced spring onions. Add half a can of drained tuna (flaked) and 2 tbsp low-calorie mayo. Toss together and serve.	An apple or a handful of berries.	A glass of your favourite tipple.
Day 78: Monday	A hearty bowl of fruit salad and a small pot of yoghurt.	A serving of Perfect Pea Soup (see page 76) with two wholemeal crackers.	Lemon-Roasted Chicken & Potatoes (see page 72) with broccoli and carrots.	A nice cuppa with semi-skimmed milk and a plain biscuit.	

12 WEEK PLAN	BREAKFAST	LUNCH	DINNER	SNACK ON...	A LITTLE OF WHAT YOU FANCY
Day 79: Tuesday	Toasted crumpet topped with slices of strawberry and a teaspoon of runny honey.	Grab a low-fat readymade chicken salad from your local store.	Grill a piece of fish (choose from cod, haddock or any other firm white fish). Serve with a crunchy salad and five to six small new potatoes.	Two pieces of fruit.	
Day 80: Wednesday	25g (1oz) porridge oats or a ready measured sachet made with semi-skimmed milk. Serve with chunks of banana.	Jacket potato with low-sugar baked beans.	Throw together a Veggie Stir-Fry (see page 90).	An orange or a small bunch of grapes.	Indulge in a small bag of your favourite crisps.
Day 81: Thursday	Two slices wholemeal toast spread thinly with Marmite; an apple.	One large slice of rye bread spread with low-fat cottage cheese.	Light Macaroni Cheese (see page 73) served with a choice of two veggies.	Fun size packet dried fruit.	
Day 82: Friday	Low-sugar baked beans on wholemeal toast.	Half an avocado, sliced, served with a handful of	Pitta Pizza (see page 71) topped with six small slices	An apple.	

12 WEEK PLAN	BREAKFAST	LUNCH	DINNER	SNACK ON...	A LITTLE OF WHAT YOU FANCY
		cooked prawns and shredded lettuce. Finish with 1 tbsp low-calorie Thousand Island dressing.	of pepperoni. Serve with a mixed salad.		
Day 83: Saturday	Half a ruby grapefruit and a small pot of low-fat yoghurt.	Spoil yourself with a Fish Finger Sarnie! Bake two fish fingers according to the directions on the package (do not fry) and serve in a wholemeal roll with sliced gherkins and a portion of homemade Skinny Chips (see page 73).	Enjoy a Salade Niçoise (see page 96).	A banana or a small bunch of grapes.	A glass of your favourite tipple.
Day 84: Sunday	Low-fat yoghurt and a piece of fruit.	Tuck into a Lean Roast Dinner (see page 90).	Sardines on a thick slice of wholemeal toast with a sliced few cherry tomatoes.	Two oatcakes or carrot sticks.	A glass of your favourite tipple.

A WORD ABOUT HUNGER

You may already be aware that often when we think we are hungry we are actually thirsty, so make sure you always drink water before grabbing some food. Now of course if you have been used to eating far too much food, the first few weeks will seem a little tough at times but I want you to stop and think about your hunger. Rate your hunger out of ten and if it's at least a seven, have a healthy snack. A big problem I used to suffer from myself was eating at the first sign of hunger when in fact I soon learnt that I could be satisfied with a 600ml (1 pint) glass of water instead. Alison Carman, my consultant nutritionist, explains that because we are living in a world where food is so readily available, it is easy to forget what that empty sensation in our stomach feels like. She suggests that experiencing hunger, especially when you first start a new way of eating, is quite normal so my message to you is to think first before rushing to the fridge! Some other tips follow:

Pack in the protein

Research shows that protein-rich foods help to improve satiety, which is the feeling of fullness. The more satiated you feel after eating, the less likely you'll be to feel hungry between meals. Eating small amounts of lean meat, chicken, fish, dairy products and eggs may help to keep you feeling fuller for longer.

Fill up on fibre

Swap all things white for brown to keep hunger at bay. This means dumping white spaghetti, cornflakes and white rice and instead opting for wholemeal bread, wholewheat pasta, wholegrain cereals and brown rice. Foods high in fibre help combat hunger because as well as taking longer to digest, they also take longer to chew and slow the speed at which you eat; this gives your brain time to register the feeling of fullness, so increasing satiety. Fibre acts like a sponge to absorb water and swells in the stomach, which helps you to feel full.

Start throwing dinner parties!

As you get more in control of your food and become expert at preparing healthier meal plans, why not show friends and family by entertaining following your new guidelines? This, of course, is a great way to showcase the new and improved you! As you do so, you can also show your guests the changes you have made in the way that you play host: show them that you take pride in your cooking by carefully placing food on the plates so that it looks appetising, make sure both cutlery and glasses are gleaming and lay the table perfectly.

Etiquette guru William Hanson believes this is a great way to reinforce the changes within ourselves and suggests weight loss isn't just about a change in the body but also a change in the way we conduct ourselves at the table. 'Show others *how* to eat and not just *what* to eat,' he advises. His tips include holding cutlery properly with a finger down the blade of the knife, keeping your elbows off the table and tucked into your sides and making sure the napkin goes on your lap as opposed to tucking it in underneath your neck. Talking of napkins, Hanson explains that you should dab your mouth delicately when you need to use one rather than using it like a face flannel. And when do you need a napkin the most? When you're eating soup, of course. Hanson recommends when eating soup, scoop it away from you to fill up the spoon and then sip it using the side of the spoon that has not gone into the bowl. But what about the wine at the table, I hear you cry? And the final Hanson rule: take small sips rather than simply glugging it back!

Mel's story

Mel was a bubbly character who had been massively overweight for most of her life and at 30, she was beginning to think that she would never meet a partner. She explained that most men did not find her attractive because she was morbidly obese and she accepted that in the real world, men were generally attracted to a slimmer woman. Mel deserved to be slimmer. She had an infectious personality, was intelligent and fun but recognised that her eating habits were not supporting the weight-loss goal she had carried for years. One of those people who had tried every diet going, she had been to weight-loss clubs, numerous boot camps and even tried specialist liquid-only diets. When we first met, Mel eloquently explained to me that restricted diets just didn't work for her and that she found it difficult to give up chocolate and her favourite takeaway treats. After I explained to Mel that I would never want her to ever give them up, she looked shocked, and like many of my clients, was initially confused.

For years, people preached to Mel that she had to deny herself the McDonald's breakfast, the tasty KFC meal and the curry houses on a Friday night to lose weight, which as you will know by now is something I strongly oppose. I explained to Mel that while we could build in these foods, we had to make sure it was all in proportion and what that meant was portion control. I outlined the 80–20 rule and she began to understand that losing weight was not going to be about denial but eating healthy foods 80 per cent of the time and the odd bit of so-called 'junk' food 20 per cent of the time.

As I continued to explain that we would now get to work on developing her meal plans, Mel grinned warmly. As well as implementing the 80–20 rule combined with a meal plan, we began a number of mind programming techniques using hypnotherapy to help her embed the 80–20 rule into her mind and gain control over food.

As the weeks passed, Mel became skilled in developing her meal plans to include treats during the week. She combined this with at least one hour's walking each night and the weight began to fall off. As she moved forward, her control over eating strengthened with the combination of the 80–20 rule and the use of self-hypnosis to keep her mind focused. It was good to see Mel's confidence with men improve and as far as I am aware, to this day she is still in the dating game and having lots of fun!

SECRET 7

MANAGE EMOTIONAL EATING

Now, this is the area where I struggled most for several years. When the stress kicked in, worries filled my mind and depression sank in deeply, culminating in panic attacks. And what was my release? Food! There were days when I would wake up and feel heavy and numb, so much so that I would find it a massive struggle to get out of bed. I would get up and go to the bathroom, look at my body in the mirror (which only made me feel worse) and my instinct was to run and hide under the duvet. If I'm honest, stress played a big part and of course the downright laziness within me, as well as the realisation that I really should have started to get to grips with things a while ago, didn't help. What I did learn was if the source of stress wasn't tackled then I would simply eat more. Furthermore, I needed to develop a contingency plan so that rather than eating more food, I would do something else. However, when it comes to emotional eating there is one thing you must do first and that is to take action.

In this chapter, I want to offer you support so that you can begin to work through the stress while at the same time eat less (but eat better) and move about more. At this point, I also want to strongly emphasise that if you suffer from depression, you should visit your GP. As someone who has taken anti-depressants in the past, I want you to know that if your doctor recommends you take them, for a short period of time or more long-term, then you should not feel ashamed, weak, embarrassed or a failure. In fact, it is often the strongest and most intelligent people who take medication to help them through difficult times. There is absolutely no shame in this and often it's the helping hand that you need.

WHY WE EAT WHEN STRESSED

When stressed, we release higher levels of the stress hormone cortisol. While cortisol has many benefits, too much of it – often brought on by excessive stress – can cause problems, including the triggering of a craving for salty and sweet foods. In fact, centuries ago it meant that we could build up on those foods that would help us get through the tough times. In those days, staple foods were frequently scarce. Of course, in our more fortunate society food is more widely available but this also means people can easily put on excess weight if they overindulge – especially on the processed foods, which are abundant and often very cheap.

In addition, when we eat food we experience a natural increase in serotonin, making us feel comforted and happier. Have you noticed how, when you feel a bit down and you unwrap a chocolate bar, you automatically begin to feel better, maybe even smile? In short, this is because your serotonin levels increase. The problem is that once the food has been eaten and the wrapper is in the bin, these levels drop once again and you may even begin to feel worse and perhaps beat yourself up for over-indulging. That's why, in this section of the book I want to encourage you to take control of what is causing the stress and to put in place a number of select strategies to help you beat stress so you eat less and eat better.

I'm now going to work through with you the main triggers of everyday stress and offer advice on how to manage them. Key stresses found by leading stress management experts, Holmes and Rahe, include:

- *Financial problems:* For example, managing a shortfall of cash, increasing your levels of debt including credit card payments, cost of children's education and impending bankruptcy.
- *Life stresses:* For example, workplace and personal stresses.
- *Relationships:* Difficulties may include constant arguments with your spouse or children, family illness, kids leaving home, etc.

MANAGING DEBT

As Mike Thomas of debtwizard.com explains there is nothing wrong with debt, provided you can manage the repayments. Unfortunately, many of us need to have some debt in order to be able to function in today's material world but when debt spirals out of control stress increases, as does the amount of comfort eating you do when you hope the debt will go away. To prevent your debt getting out of hand, apply the following ground rules:

- Never borrow more than you can afford. Yes it's obvious, but so often completely ignored!
- Put together a budget to make sure you live within your means.
- If you have a problem re-paying a loan, discuss this with the company involved or a financial advisor sooner rather than later – leaving it will only make matters worse.
- Borrowing can be very expensive so think hard before you commit yourself to a loan, particularly credit cards. Consider the monthly repayments and check the total amount that you will have to pay back, including interest and all administration charges. Be aware that any insurance taken out to protect your payments on a loan can be expensive, too.
- Sometimes it's better to 'save to spend' rather than 'borrow to spend'.
- If you have a mortgage, fixing it on a low interest rate may be useful.
- When you're thinking of buying an item, ask yourself, 'How am I going to pay for this?' and 'What's the cheapest way of doing this?' Look for interest-free deals.
- It's not a race to see who can reach the credit card limit first! Make your card work for you by settling the balance every month to avoid any additional costs, but do arrange additional benefits such as purchase protection and air miles.
- Don't need it or can't afford it? Don't buy it!

A WORD ABOUT BUSINESS DEBT

If you run your own business, you may also be concerned about business debt. The emotional pressure this brings as demand for a particular product or service drops is often immense and can cause the highest-flying entrepreneur to turn to food for comfort. When it comes to dealing with business debt issues, it is vitally important that you seek advice and know what your options are. If things get difficult, the usual route is for a business to enter into an arrangement with its creditors and trade out of the debt over a number of years. This is known as an Individual Voluntary Arrangement (IVA) for a sole trader and Company Voluntary Arrangement (CVA) for limited companies. Another option is the Administration Order, which ring-fences all current debts while a rescue package is put in place. If all else fails, it's personal bankruptcy for the sole trader and liquidation for a limited company.

What's clear is that if debt looks as if it's becoming an issue, seek advice at the earliest opportunity – normally from a chartered accountant who is also a licensed Insolvency Practitioner (IP). Do not ignore the signs in the hope that it will all just go away. Also, bear in mind that it is a criminal offence for a director of a limited company to continue trading while insolvent, so start out on the right footing. You can find contact details of licensed Insolvency Practitioners at http://www.insolvencydirect.bis.gov.uk/fip1.

It is also important to remember that you have nothing to be ashamed of as you deal with business debt. We live in an uncertain world where economic growth in many parts of the economy is stagnant so don't beat yourself up: remember, you're not the only one and there is support out there.

THE MIKE THOMAS FIVE-POINT PLAN

Anyone who has experienced debt problems will tell you what a nightmare it can be. Often it's the frustration and stress in not knowing where to start, what information is required of you and who to contact. With years of experience, moneywise Mike Thomas helps consumers overcome their debt issues and has put together the following plan. Not only will you regain control of your debts but more importantly, you'll regain control of your life!

1. Find out what you owe and to whom

Get together all your recent credit and store card statements, any loan agreements and bank statements and draw up a list for each of the following:

- Those in your name only.
- Those in your partner's name only (if applicable) and those in joint names, i.e. your name and someone else's (if applicable).

Don't forget to list all forms of borrowing and remember to include any from family and friends, payday and doorstep loans. You then need to identify which loans are secured (such as a mortgage on a property or a hire purchase loan on a vehicle) and those classed as priority debts, then any other priority creditors/lenders, such as utilities and council tax. Now make a separate list of your unsecured creditors/lenders, such as personal loans, credit and store cards. It's important to remember that if you don't pay secured creditors then you may lose security (your house, for example) and if you don't pay priority creditors such as your electricity or gas provider, you may forfeit the services they provide.

2. What are you worth? Let's see what assets you have

An asset could be your house, even if the property is mortgaged. To work out the interest you have in the property, simply take any outstanding mortgage away from the value of your home. For example, if the house is in your name only and your mortgage debt stands at £70,000 and your house is valued at around £100,000, then your asset is worth £30,000. However, if the mortgage is shared with a partner, then the £30,000 is divided between the two of you and you each have an asset worth £15,000. Of course assets can be other items of worth, such as jewellery, antiques, shares, etc.

3. Establish how much you can really afford to pay your creditors

You now need to work out your total family income – this will include salary/wages, tax credits, benefits, etc. Your next list needs to be your outgoings: what you spend each week/month on food, clothing, utilities and transport, etc., including payments to secured creditors but not those unsecured ones. Once you have taken your outgoings away from your income you will be left with a figure known in financial circles as 'disposable income' (DI). The amount of DI will help you assess your options when it comes to dealing with creditors as it clearly shows what you can really afford to pay towards your debts. All this information is essential when seeking advice on the way forward.

4. Talk to your creditors/lenders

Because many consumers are confused, worried or even embarrassed about speaking to their creditors/lenders often they will just ignore letters and phone calls about their debt situation. If you fail to make payments to your creditors and don't communicate with them at all, they will regard you as someone who won't pay rather than a person who can't pay. This leaves them with little option but to take legal action against you to recover their losses. When you make contact, they will ask for the information you have prepared in steps one to three above and only then will they be able to make a decision on how best to help you. Above all, be realistic and accept there is a problem and it will only go away if you do something about it.

5. Get that important advice

Mike Thomas believes that it can be better to seek professional advice before speaking to your creditors/ lenders as this ensures you have all the right information to hand and are already aware of bankruptcy, IVA/CVA trade outs, Debt Relief Orders (DRO) and debt repayment programme options available to you. This also avoids you being talked into doing something unsuited to your financial situation. Advice is available from various debt charities or commercial firms and both have advantages and disadvantages. For example, the charities are currently swamped with enquiries and are largely funded by creditors, which some believe influences the advice being given. However, you do not pay fees for their services. With a commercial firm you will pay fees, but they will represent you and not the creditors. Many firms are also able to offer a better level of service that the charities – but make sure you check out the company thoroughly because some 'debt management' firms are not worth the money. You will find that debtwizard.com lists both types of organisation and it's up to you, the consumer, to decide what best suits your needs.

One final note: stay positive and don't give up

If a creditor or lender refuses your offer of repayment, or to stop the interest charges you are incurring on top of your debt, reaffirm your efforts. Get them to give up – and not you! Never borrow more money to pay off your creditors, unless you have been professionally advised to do so. Don't be afraid to seek specialist help and advice – and don't ignore the problem either! Hoping it will just go away is not the answer. Just remember not to be intimidated, threatened or bullied into making offers or promises that you know you won't be able to keep. It's not a crime to be in debt, so insist you are treated fairly and with respect.

MANAGING GENERAL STRESS

Without some pressures in life we wouldn't function: we all need some stimulation and pressure is what drives us to live life and take on new challenges. In fact, pressure can make your work more satisfying and help you meet your objectives but it's when pressure becomes too much to handle that stress starts to kick in. Stress management is therefore about taking action to do something to manage the pressure so that it doesn't boil over.

Of course stress is different for everyone and often depends on your personality and the perceptions that different people hold. For example, for one person, being stuck in a traffic jam might be perceived as something they have no control over and so they may as well relax, while another might regard it as a complete nightmare and immediately suffer symptoms of stress. Can you guess what many of the latter do? You've got it – they reach for food! So, what are the symptoms of stress? They vary greatly but some may include:

• Headaches.
• Tense muscles.
• Irritable Bowel Syndrome (IBS).
• Insomnia and other sleep problems.
• Skin rashes and break-outs.
• Raised heart rate.
• Sense of humour failure.
• Sweating.
• Dizziness and blurred vision.
• Anger and outbursts.
• Reduced confidence.
• Problems in concentrating.
• Loss of libido.
• Lack of motivation.
• Self-doubt.

It's when we begin to experience the above (and sometimes a combination of symptoms) that we need to take action to proactively manage ourselves and bring our life pressures down to a more realistic level. Of course, this can be tough at times because many things are out of our control – for example, the hours we work, our colleagues, how badly our favourite football team is performing, etc. However, without some form of action things can get a whole lot worse and lead to rapid weight gain, serious health problems, even death.

MANAGING STRESS AT WORK

If the source of your stress is at work, there a number of things you can do. First, take steps to help yourself – for example, making sure your working environment is as safe, relaxed and comfortable as possible. To do this, ensure you have good lighting, your chair is at a comfortable height and a bowl of fruit is on hand rather than sugary or fatty alternatives. Try to also control your hours and while this can be tricky in these recessionary times, don't be embarrassed to ask about flexible working hours as many employers now offer this facility.

It may be the case that you are stressed at work because you feel you are being bullied or harassed. If this is the case, find out if your employer has any policies in these areas and don't be afraid to speak in confidence to the human resources department. Maybe you find stress at work hard to handle. If so, implement your own strategy for dealing with it, such as exercising before and after work, which will help release feel-good endorphins. Look for a new hobby or interest to take your mind off things – personally, I always find talking it over with good friends really helps and it's much better than chewing on junk food. Above all, don't be too hard on yourself: remember, taking action to reduce stress at work is the best way forward. If it's the job itself, think about reassessing your choice of work or moving to a different employer, but do take immediate action to get on the career path you really want. It doesn't have to be a big step, just something small, such as researching the career itself and identifying what you need to do to get there. Or it could be something major that you've had in the back of your mind but kept putting off, such as starting your own business.

Stress often exists when we do nothing. Taking action immediately helps to reduce stress because you feel something is happening – often it's down to managing your own perception of what's causing the stress, being able to get things into perspective and learning to relax more. Sometimes all you need to do is take a step back from your situation: try and view your situation as others might do and this can provide a whole new perspective. More than likely it will also take away some, if not all, of the stressful burden.

PRACTICE RELAXATION

There are numerous ways to relax but one of the best is something I teach many of my clients: self-induced relaxation. Follow the stages below and practice the technique. It can act as a highly effective daily chill-out and once you get the hang of it, this may become something you can do easily and also look forward to.

- Find somewhere comfortable where it is safe, warm and as distraction-free as possible. Sit upright in your seat and place your hands on your thighs.
- Now close your eyes and think of a peaceful scene. This can be somewhere you know well or even a fantasy place. Allow yourself to enjoy that scene for a couple of minutes as you breathe deeply. Notice how you begin to calm down and also how you are able to breathe out the stress.
- Mentally count down from ten to one on every other out-breath. As you do so, imagine yourself sinking down into a wonderful state of relaxation.

If you hear outside noises, blend them into the process by telling yourself the noises help you relax even more deeply because you know you're safe and sound as you relax. It's that very familiar feeling you get when you nod off to sleep at night.

- Once you've counted down from ten to one allow yourself to notice the peaceful and relaxing scene in detail. Pay attention to what you see, hear and feel; tell yourself anything unimportant can fall away. This will help you become fully associated with the peaceful scene.

- Remain in your peaceful scene for as long as you like. Keep breathing freely and notice the tension melt away as you breathe out.

- Once you are ready to wake up, all you need to do is count from one to ten and on the count of ten, open your eyes. Tell yourself as soon as you reach number eight, any feelings of numbness and heaviness will have completely disappeared and that you will wake up feeling refreshed and ready to enjoy the rest of your day.

CONSIDER COMPLEMENTARY TECHNIQUES

Complementary support available outside the realms of traditional medicine can be very effective indeed. The techniques may help to restore the body's balance allowing it to cope with the everyday stresses life throws at us. Complementary techniques can also boost the immune system, help alleviate toxins, relieve pain, improve circulation and establish better sleep patterns and also help you to achieve a deep state of relaxation. They may also be used to target a specific health problem and act as a preventative measure for certain illnesses. If you want to treat yourself, there are some wonderful complementary therapies out there. The ones I recommend include acupuncture, reflexology and aromatherapy. If this is your bag, always check the practitioner's experience and that they are suitably accredited; also, make sure there are no contra-indications (conditions or ailments you suffer from) that could mean the therapy would be unsuitable for you (a professional practitioner will be able to advise you on this).

REDUCE DEPRESSION

As someone who has suffered from periods of depression, I myself know only too well how debilitating this can be. I always advocate visiting your GP if you feel depressed, if only to talk things over. Those suffering from depression often report symptoms such as feelings of worthlessness, hollowness and emptiness. During my darkest days, I would feel apathetic and stay in bed a lot of the time with curtains drawn. If you are at that stage, I would urge you to seek medical intervention via your GP. When we are depressed stress hormones such as cortisol are higher and levels of serotonin (which lift our mood) can be lower.

Working with your GP or specialist counsellor, you can develop a plan to reduce some of the pressures you have in life; you will also learn how to stimulate your mood through activities such as increasing your level of exercise and start to believe in yourself when you make small achievements. It's important to avoid role conflict – by this I mean trying to be something you are not to try and please others or get a sense of acceptance. A classic example might be someone who has been promoted into a management or leadership role at work but does not have the necessary skills to carry this through and subsequently becomes stressed by the burden and expectations placed on them. If this is your situation, think about the person you really are and what you can do, not just what others expect you to be.

Trying to be something you are not only increases the pressure within and can lead to serious depressive illness. Trust me, I know! For several years I tried to be what society expected of me and guess what that resulted in? The day I told myself that I was going to be what I wanted to be was the day I found liberation in my own skin. Beforehand, I was trying to be something that didn't feel right, didn't appear right and certainly didn't look right (to me and others). Let yourself be who you want to be irrespective of other people. Remember, in general most of us believe you have only one life and so you need to make the most of it and not live your life for other people: give yourself permission to be who you truly are.

ACCEPT THE THINGS YOU CANNOT CHANGE

Some stressful situations will be unavoidable. For example, in my own case running a business when a recession hits can become stressful at times, but I have to accept there is nothing I can do about it. It has taken a while but I find the best way to deal with life stresses that I cannot change is to accept things as they are. Of course this is easier said than done, but in the long run it's much easier than trying to fight it and allowing myself to get into an unhealthy emotional and physical state.

Where possible, don't try and control the uncontrollable, such as the behaviour of others. When faced with difficult personalities, concentrate on what you can change, such as your own reaction to them. With situations that you have no control over, such as the loss of a loved one, it's important to share your feelings and talk things through. Avoid bottling your feelings up and instead express them to someone because this will help to relieve the stress. It's really important to remember that if you cannot change the stress, try and change yourself by changing your attitude and perception.

Take Simon, for example. He came to see me and explained that people around him were stressing him out at work and also the business he worked in was undergoing rapid change. Simon had to realise there was nothing he could do about this stressful situation, but there *was* something he could do about himself. Eventually, he learnt how to reframe this particular problem and instead of seeing all the negatives of the change decided to view it from a more positive perspective. He also looked at the bigger picture and asked himself how he could benefit in the long run rather than focusing his mind on what he was losing. Encouraging Simon to focus more on the positives also helped him to look at what else he had so that he could appreciate how good life actually was. It was these strategies that helped him keep it all in perspective.

SEIZE CONTROL OF UNNECESSARY STRESS

While there are many stresses we cannot avoid, there are some that we can and often these are the ones that may encourage you to over-eat to feel a bit better. Here are some of the stressful situations we can remove from our daily lives by taking a few simple actions:

- Deliberately take yourself away from people who stress you out. This can include friends who are good at making you feel down and negative following their draining conversations. Don't feel guilty about ignoring their calls or saying no to them when they make demands on your time and emotional resources. In fact, take the major step of deleting them from your life altogether if it's really that bad.

- Remove stress by turning off the TV if it's just bad news or decide to read only the positive news in the newspaper. Avoid everyday arguments – for example, religion or politics – if you find they trigger anger and anxiety in you. Such things can be bad for your blood pressure!

USE PRACTICAL STRESSBUSTERS

There's nothing better than identifying a few techniques that work for you on an everyday level. Listed below in no particular order is my Top 20:

1. Have a long soak in the bath (make sure you will not be distracted).
2. Go for a good long walk, alone or with a friend or partner.
3. Use aromatherapy oils on the pillow at night. I always use lavender oil. However, make sure you read the instructions carefully when using aromatherapy oils as they are not suitable for everyone.
4. Have a good laugh watching one of your favourite comedies.

5. Put on some music that helps you to completely chill out.
6. Read a good book that takes you away from everyday life.
7. Enjoy some good-quality sex, but don't light up a cigarette afterwards!
8. Treat yourself to a massage or reflexology.
9. Have a good long chat with a close friend and let it all out.
10. Play with your pets or borrow a neighbour's dog and take it for a walk.
11. Go to the gym and have a good workout.
12. Write down your feelings in a journal.
13. Practice self-induced relaxation (see page 134).
14. Get a punch-bag and use this to let out any pent-up anger.
15. Allow yourself to be pampered by taking a short spa break.
16. Set some stretching goals to stimulate your mind and drive your passion for doing something other than sitting on the couch.
17. Take up a new hobby or interest that excites you.
18. Do something for fun, such as going to an open-air concert with friends.
19. De-clutter the house so that it's out with the old and in with the new.
20. Do something exciting that involves the family, lets you have a good laugh and lets your inner child run free.

CONQUERING PANIC ATTACKS

As I mentioned at the beginning of this book, panic attacks were the driving force behind my own major life change and the reason why I got to grips with losing weight. Panic attacks entered my life at a time when I was too fat and under way too much stress, so much so that my ability to cope with the stress and weight gain was seemingly out of reach. Inside, I felt confused, agitated, shaky and let's face it, pretty weak; life had become too much and the only comfort to cushion me from the panic attacks I suffered was food. Oh yes, I would eat lots, and I mean *lots*! I would think nothing of stuffing myself with a couple of packets of biscuits and sometimes I would mix them with ice cream! *Ice cream?* I hear you shriek, but how could a weight-loss motivator like me binge eat? The answer is very simple: natural human responses to stress is fight or flight, so I fled away from dealing with my life pressures and found solace in food and isolation.

If you are someone else who suffers from panic attacks I want to give you hope, confidence and optimism that things really can get better and that in time you will conquer the vicious circle that these debilitating panic attacks can get you into. The symptoms of panic attacks differ from person to person. For some, it's a shortness of breath and an inability to breathe, while others feel faint and this can lead to sweating, trembling and shaking. The first thing I want you to know is that panic attacks are actually more common than you might imagine. As someone who treats panic attacks, I can tell you that people of all ages and backgrounds suffer from them and you have no reason to feel ashamed or embarrassed if you happen to be one of them.

A panic attack occurs when adrenaline is released into your bloodstream and a message of fear sends a signal to the adrenal glands that there's an emergency. The adrenaline causes the body to pump extra blood, which in turn gets pumped into the major muscles to increase strength in your arms and your ability to run fast: fight or flight. This extra blood also shoots into your brain, giving you the heightened ability to respond to an emergency. Research suggests that it takes a few minutes from the time your brain sends the emergency signal until your body is full of adrenaline, with this extra blood in your arm and leg muscles, as well as your brain. During those few minutes, your heart will be pumping harder and extra blood flows through your body. If your adrenal glands continue to get an emergency message, they will continue to release additional adrenaline. It's when your brain stops signalling an emergency that your adrenal glands hold the adrenaline instead of releasing it. However, there are some techniques to help prevent panic attacks. Consider the following ideas:

- Avoid fighting the panic: The more you try and fight it, the greater the intensity of the panic attack. Sounds crazy I know, but start welcoming them in! Most probably you will find the attacks lessen in intensity.
- Learn to calm yourself: Use deep breathing to help your mind reach a state of calm.
- Interrupt the panic driving thoughts by shouting the word STOP loudly inside your head. Alternatively, if you find certain situations trigger panic, sing a nursery rhyme loudly inside your head. This helps to interrupt the emergency

message that the brain is sending to your adrenal glands.

- Reframe your thoughts: Instead of saying to yourself, 'Oh, now my heart is pounding and I think I'm going to have a heart attack!' say: 'The fear I am carrying right now is making my heart pound faster but that's okay because I know I am safe.' Or rather than saying, 'Oh no, here I go again, I feel *awful*!' say to yourself, 'Here we go again, but I have experienced it lots of times now and I know that I'm safe and nothing bad is going to happen to me.'

- Try distraction techniques: There are a number of different distraction techniques that will help refocus your mind so that the panic attack is eliminated. Here, I offer you four techniques – doing them all at the same time is most productive! The first technique is the 'counting distraction', where you count down from 100 as quickly as possible and then repeat it. The second technique is to take yourself away to splash cold water over your face. This triggers what is known as a 'dive reflex' and encourages the brain to instruct your body to 'go slow'. The third technique for you to try is to use a physical, visual and audio stimulus, such as turning on the TV to watch a riotous comedy, or do something that makes you happy – for example, singing loudly to your favourite music. If you are in an appropriate place, you might also dance very physically to the music to distract your thoughts (the mind will concentrate on moving the body), as well as singing out loud.

Remember, you can do anything that works for you so long as it distracts your mind from anxiety. The final distraction is one that I was taught during my training in hypnotherapy: shake your hands and clench your fists. This helps to remove the adrenaline build-up and begins to calm you.

• Do visit your GP if you suffer regular panic attacks and consider advice from a certified clinical hypnotherapist. I regularly post information and advice about anxiety and panic attacks, so please visit my website: www.thestevemillerplan.com.

MANAGING YOUR RELATIONSHIPS

The relationship with yourself

Relationship coach Jackie Walker suggests that developing a relationship with yourself is just like being on an aeroplane when you are told to put on your oxygen mask in case of emergency before putting on anyone else's. In other words, you have to love yourself before being able to pass love on. This can be very difficult if you are overweight and it might be that you are in a Catch-22 situation where your relationship isn't right and that's your excuse for over-eating.

Jackie claims there is nothing more exhausting than being in conflict with your inner self and suggests that it's essential to accept fallibility and to recognise that there is no such thing as perfection. And she's right: you are perfect because you're *you*! Jackie explains that if instead of constantly noticing the gap between where you are now and where you want to be, you start going about life wanting what you have then you will probably find things start to look a little more positive. In allowing the pressure to be taken off, not only will you allow yourself to accept yourself more but also allows yourself to be at peace within. It's also a crucial step for many in breaking that over-eating cycle, which allows them to naturally reduce food cravings, take up more exercise and shed the pounds.

Relationships with the kids

If you have kids, then they are your world but there can be no doubting that at times parents can struggle with holding down a workable solid relationship with their offspring. Sue Atkins is a renowned expert on parenting and has published several books on the topic. She explains that being a parent is a twenty-four hours of the day, seven days of the week and fifty-two weeks of the year job and because kids don't come with a handbook, parenting can feel very overwhelming, challenging and tiring at times. Sue has a number of tips to help parents be the best they can and this in turn allows them to relax, knowing they are doing their best and also helps them to develop a solid relationship with their kids. Talking with Sue, I picked up a number of down-to-earth practical strategies, as listed below:

- Children spell love T-I-M-E so get involved in your child's life by playing with them, talking with them and eating with them every day.
- Read to your child for 15 minutes each day and enjoy discussing the stories and themes to create a love of learning with them.
- Snuggle up at bedtime and enjoy the closeness of bonding over reading and sharing a book together.

This builds vocabulary in addition to closeness and your child will also do well at school since they will become confident at reading with an active imagination.

- Talk to your child with the television off. One simple way to communicate with your youngster is to sit down and enjoy a healthy meal together and have fun chatting about both your days. Don't nag them to eat their broccoli or to hold their knife and fork properly! Make it all about relaxing, chatting and having fun together.
- Make sure you are a positive role model yourself in the way you view life and be aware of the words you use, your tone of voice and your body language, as children learn from you all the time. Adopt a positive, upbeat attitude and watch your child flourish.
- Scold less, praise more and watch your child's self-esteem blossom. Deliberately look for what your child gets right and praise them specifically and generously, then watch your child do even more to please you.
- Be consistent in your discipline. Grab a pen and paper and fold it in half on one side, then write down some simple rules that you want your kids to follow. On the other side write down a list of things that are unacceptable to you. Next, write down the consequences if your child doesn't do as he is told. Now you have a simple framework to work from. Sit down and have a chat about these rules to make sure your kids know what they are and what will happen if they break them. Keep it

simple and watch your life get easier. Don't go for an approach that gives a short-term gain but builds up a long-term nightmare: remember the bigger picture because families who have simple rules and are consistent have less stress and better relationships.

- Listen first, talk later. Listening makes children feel valued, heard and understood. It also makes them feel important. By listening properly to your kids, you help them find their own answers; they also let off steam in this way. You might even get to ask the odd great question and your child may start to see things from a different perspective. So turn off the TV, put down the newspaper and stop peeling the potatoes! Look your child in the eye, turn your heart to their heart and give them your full attention. Listen with genuine interest and really pay attention to what they're telling you. Keep an open mind and don't judge or interrupt – you know how frustrating it is when someone interrupts you, or half listens, or just says, 'aha' every now and again. Your kids deserve better and remember, you have two ears and only one mouth for a reason!

- Be loving. Ignore the old wives' tale that hugging, holding or telling your kids that you love them is spoiling them. You can never be too loving! I have never met a child who was worse off because their parents loved them too much. Hug them, tickle them, play with them and find time to listen to them – it builds memories that last a lifetime.

Coping with sick relatives or loved ones

Learning how to manage a relationship with a loved one or a relative who is suffering from an ongoing illness can be challenging – and I know only too well how this can lead you to make food your best friend! At times, food may seem the only thing that will get you through the day. As you look after your loved one, it's important to listen to their concerns and for them to know you are there for them and to help meet their needs, but remember you have to look after yourself, too. Frequently it's the person giving care who becomes ill as they do their best to carry out what they feel is their nursing responsibility. Of course, it's important to care but I want you to know that you must care for yourself as well – and without feeling guilty. It's that guilt that affects your ability to look after yourself, so let it go! After all, what use will you be if you become ill, too?

Learn to be assertive because then you will get the support you need and your needs will also be met. There is nothing wrong with asking for help and making requests to other people. DO NOT FEEL GUILTY! When dealing with the NHS, make sure you ask for the support of a nurse, if needed and if you have an important appointment with the doctor, prepare questions in advance so that it meets your needs. Never see yourself as second rate to those who wear the uniforms: they are there to serve you, not the other way round! You may want to take someone with you when you visit the medics; they can help you ask uncomfortable questions and be there to put an arm around you, if needed. Be assertive and use the 'I' statement explaining what it is you need to start moving forward otherwise you believe the health of your loved one or relative will suffer.

Rob Harris, author of *A Caregivers Story – We Are In This Together*, writes from the heart about how he cares for his wife, who had cancer. He explains that as a new caregiver it is natural to worry and that it is the fear of the unknown and the stress induced when questioning your ability to handle something with which you are unfamiliar, especially when it concerns the present and the future. By nature, Rob was a worrier and as his wife became seriously ill, he worried even more. In fact, he would worry to such a degree that he was making himself nauseous on a daily basis. He explains that while his wife was handling her cancer in a positive and proactive fashion, he worried enough for the both of them. In his book, he now looks back and asks a number of questions: What did it do for her? What did it do for me? What did it do for our friends and family members? Rob concludes his pent-up state caused them to worry about him! In being a caregiver to his wife, he had to develop a number of strategies to help eliminate the anxiety and pressure of being a caregiver.

Rob adopted the phrase, 'It is what it is'. While some may disagree, this phrase helped him to focus on the fact that his wife was ill and there was nothing he could do to eradicate the cancer from her system. Therefore, he had to accept the fact that his role was one of support and worrying about her would not be supportive; catering to her needs would be a more positive alternative. Rob incorporated laughter, *lots* of laughter, into his day with his wife. If they received bad news, he allowed himself only an hour to worry about it. Afterwards, he compartmentalised his concerns and tried his best to ignore the emotional symptoms accompanying it. Vigorous exercise helped a great deal as it dissolved much of the pent-up energy created by worrying; he also listened to his favourite music when his wife slept, socialised with happy, positive people and avoided those with a doom and gloom attitude. Rob tried to spend as much time as possible with his loved ones and also played with his pets.

Of course none of these tips will change your set of circumstances but they might help you to cope with whatever it is you are facing. Rob explains that worry is a thought – nothing more, nothing less – and the issues themselves will not change, only the way in which you deal with them. More details on Rob's story can be found at www.robcares.com.

In short, combine the stress management techniques described in this book with Rob's advice and always look after your own needs. Don't feel bad about taking time out, enjoying the company of friends or even some leisure activity. If the pressure becomes too much, consider counselling or hypnotherapy to help manage the stress you are experiencing. And remember, you should NEVER feel guilty!

Managing binge eating

If you are one of those people who over-eats on a regular basis and it has become an uncontrollable habit, you may be suffering from binge eating. Individuals who binge are compulsive overeaters and this simply makes them feel worse. In fact, binge eating disorder is more common than bulimia and anorexia and it affects both men and women.

Nevertheless, the good news is that binge eating can be treated and you can also learn how to control it. It is characterised by compulsive overeating, where people eat huge amounts of food, all the while feeling out of control and incapable of stopping. Binges can last around two hours but there are some sufferers who eat on and off all day, even when they're not hungry. A binge eater may also gorge their food so fast that they fail to taste or even be aware of what they are eating. However, unlike bulimics, they will not attempt to make themselves sick afterwards. Instead, they feel guilty and depressed about the amount of food they have consumed. Symptoms can include:

- Being unable to stop eating or control what they are eating.
- Quickly consuming large amounts of food without even noticing it.
- Eating even when full.
- Hiding or piling up food to eat later in secret, such as under a pillow in the bedroom.
- Eating normally around others, but gorging alone.
- Throughout the day eating continuously with no meal plans at all.
- Feeling ashamed about how much they have eaten.
- A numb sensation while bingeing, as if they're not really there or they're on autopilot.
- Never satisfied, no matter how much is eaten.
- Desperately wanting to control their weight.

Binge eating is a bit like having an addiction to food, where food acts as the drug. Unlike hard drugs, though, you still need to eat something and so going cold turkey can be difficult. However, there is the exception with certain types of food and drink, the ones you know are not good for you and can therefore banish from the kitchen. If you think you might be suffering from binge eating, then you need to develop a healthier relationship with food and one where food satisfies nutritional needs as opposed to emotional ones. To help with this, follow the secrets that work for you within this book. Working with a registered clinical hypnotherapist is something you may also like to consider as this can be extremely useful in treating such a disorder.

Susan's story

Susan was a 44-year-old business executive responsible for sales and marketing and at 121 kilos (19 stone), she was vastly overweight. Holding down a demanding job meant that she often experienced stress. She understood that stress was the key reason why she ate too much because it gave her that feel-good factor, which she needed to get through the pressure of work. For Susan, this was a Catch-22 situation because she would comfort eat and then beat herself up for being so fat. Susan believed that her weight was also affecting her ability to get results: she felt her clients judged her negatively as she grew fatter.

Working with Susan, it was obvious that we needed to build a stress management strategy to help her control the pressure more constructively. Using food as the crutch was unproductive from both a health and confidence perspective. I worked with Susan over just two sessions and she developed the following plan of action:

Daily stress control
- Each evening practice self hypnosis at home to help programme a relaxed and calm mind.
- Increase levels of personal assertion, professionally and personally.
- Take yourself away from the stress for just five minutes and practice relaxation.
- Eat healthier foods such as fruit and raw vegetables during the day.
- Implement the 80–20 Plan to help improve general nutrition.

Weekly stress control
- Take one night out each week to have fun with friends or family.
- Swim three times a week to help burn off the stress and get fitter.
- Reflect on the week and take action as needed to improve further.

Susan eventually went on to lose a total of five stone in weight, and I put this down to her ability to manage stress more effectively.

John's story

John was a young guy who came to see me because he was eating too much due to the panic attacks he was suffering. Having experienced panic attacks myself, I was only too aware of the effect these monsters can have on people. John was a genuine, well-mannered guy, who explained that when he graduated and started his first job he lost all his confidence and began to notice he was suffering from panic attacks. The panic attacks would come from nowhere and he now found himself anxious about the next one. Food was the only comfort for John, as he explained how he would get home from work at night and enjoy as much food as possible. This would usually include cakes, crisps, chocolate bars and fried foods. No wonder he gained 19 kilos (3 stone) in six months! I explained to John that to control his eating meant we first had to control the panic attacks. Following this, I developed a five-stage plan to manage his panic attacks, as described below:

- *Session One*: A full case history was taken before conducting a session of hypnotherapy to help John relax and realise he could be calm again.
- *Session Two*: In this second session, I delivered hypnotherapy designed to remove the trigger of the anxiety/panic.
- *Session Three*: During the third session of hypnotherapy, I helped John

begin to take back the control, which helped to restore a calm and focused mind as well as building his confidence.

- *Session Four.* At the fourth session, I used hypnotherapy to help John release anxiety about anxiety. This was very important because he was spending much of his day worried about the next panic attack.
- *Session Five*: In the final session, I installed further confidence into John's mind to help him move forward into the future free from panic and anxiety.

John told me that he found his panic attacks would often intensify among crowds. For example, he could not go to the cinema or see his favourite bands because the panic attacks would kick in. With this in mind, I agreed to go to a concert with him. Having done some hypnotherapy, John reported that he felt more in control and although he still experienced a feeling of anxiety, it was much less intense. In effect, he had managed to cool down his nervous system, increase his confidence and feel more relaxed for such situations.

John's story is an example where being overweight is triggered by an underlying condition, which in this case was anxiety. His example, I hope, will be an inspiration to those of you who are struggling with anxiety and panic attacks, as I once did. With carefully tailored support, they can be overcome. John is now enjoying a life that is panic-free and is successfully reducing his weight. He is no longer chained to the house as he used to be and instead enjoys playing football, spending time with his new girlfriend and being able to enjoy all the things that panic attacks used to prevent him from doing.

SECRET 8

PROGRAM YOUR MIND

When losing and controlling weight there can be no doubt that understanding how programming your mind can help develop new eating and lifestyle habits is essential. But why is it so important? Well, first of all it's vital to know how the human mind functions so that you are aware of how to influence your thoughts to help you lose weight. It has long been agreed that our mind is split into two distinct areas, namely the 'conscious' and 'unconscious' (sometimes the 'unconscious' may be referred to as the 'subconscious', although both terms mean the same). So, what is the difference between the conscious and subconscious mind?

Our conscious mind provides 'the what's going on now' element. In other words, it consists of the thoughts we are aware of at any given moment in time. So, as you read these words right now, you are consciously aware of each one of them at the same time as being aware of the environment around you: for example, the sun shining through the window, or if you are sipping a cup of tea or coffee, you will be aware of the taste and sensation of drinking something hot. You are also aware of others around you impacting on the physical environment. In essence, it is an awareness of the here and now. I often describe the human mind to my clients as being very much like an iceberg. Usually we only see a very small tip of an iceberg above the surface of the water while the bulk lies beneath the waves. The mind may be viewed in the same way, with the conscious mind acting as the tip of the iceberg and the unconscious – which is the main part of the mind – hidden beneath the surface, but influencing everything that's going on.

The unconscious mind comprises everything we know but are not actually aware of, i.e. *consciously* aware of. It holds all we have learnt – our experiences, memories, skills and the core beliefs and attitudes we hold about ourselves. The unconscious mind is also in control of automatic physical functions, including our breathing and heart rate; it controls our reactions to events and our response to stress, too. This is because your unconscious mind knows you best and has been programmed by the thoughts you have offered it. From all this, you'll know that it's the crucial part of the mind that can put you back in control of your body image, weight gain and weight loss.

Every thought you have gets logged in your unconscious mind. If, in the past, you have constantly told yourself that losing weight is difficult, then your unconscious mind will have accepted that belief. And if you have always pictured yourself fat, your unconscious mind will hold that image of you as the norm. This is because your unconscious mind accepts every single thing you tell it; whether by what you say to yourself or the pictures you paint in your mind. So, get your 'self' talk back on track to affirm the positives (for example, 'I *can* lose weight') and picture yourself slim and happy to lose weight effectively.

Your conscious and unconscious minds work in very different ways. Unlike the unconscious, the conscious mind is analytical and critical. The conscious mind is logical, sequential, judgemental and rational too, whereas the unconscious is more intuitive and involved in emotions and feelings. Sometimes there is a conflict between the conscious and unconscious mind: your conscious may want to follow one course of action whereas the unconscious may want to do the opposite. So, you may be consciously telling yourself not to stop and look in the bakery window at all the delicious fresh cakes, but your unconscious remembers what a bad time you've been having, so you think sod it and wolf down a couple of chocolate éclairs!

The reason for this is that the unconscious may be rooted in an emotional reason for taking a different course of behaviour. In these circumstances, it is normally the unconscious that wins because emotion is far stronger than logic. Let's take someone who is desperately trying to lose weight but always struggles. While they may consciously think of really strong reasons to lose weight, their unconscious mind struggles to agree because they have consistently told themselves that it's harder now they are older, or perhaps they continue to hold images of themselves as being fat and depressed. However, if they decide to work at this on both a conscious and unconscious level, then changing eating and lifestyle habits for the long haul will be far more conducive to long-term weight loss and weight control. At this point, I want you to remember that it's the unconscious mind that wins because of the emotional pull it has over logic. Your unconscious is a bit like the hard drive on a computer: we install programs on it, leave files on it and alter the way it functions. Yes, what we tell it, it instantly accepts!

WORKING WITH YOUR UNCONSCIOUS MIND

So, having learnt that the unconscious is the part of the mind you need to program to lose weight, you are probably wondering how to work with it so that it supports your immediate goal to shed weight and keep it under control in the long-term. If behaviour is controlled by your unconscious, of course it's going to be helpful to access this in order to begin re-programming.

What I will do in this chapter is offer you a three-week plan to help you communicate directly with your unconscious mind: you can program it for your benefit so that you lose weight and will be confident about keeping it off. Excited? You should be! Yes, you will be making your unconscious conscious so that you can begin taking greater control of your eating habits and life in general. You will actually be hypnotising yourself into shedding the pounds, all the while knowing you have the most powerful weight-loss tool there is inside you at all times: your brain.

USING SELF-HYPNOSIS

Self-hypnosis helps you gain greater access to your unconscious mind. Using self-hypnosis, your conscious mind will become relaxed and this allows you to communicate effectively and directly with your unconscious mind. Your conscious mind therefore becomes sleepy so that it doesn't interfere critically with what you want to do. Think of it as being a bit like a three-way conversation at home. Take a scenario where Dad is the one who always critically examines everything his son says to his wife but when Dad is asleep, the conversation between mother and son flows more effectively. In self-hypnosis it is possible to communicate directly to your unconscious mind and persuade it to do something for you. Indeed, there are a number of ways to program your unconscious to do what you want it to do, all of which are described in this chapter. This might sound like a radical process to some of you but trust me, it will allow you to re-programme your mind so that you stop being a slave to food.

By following my advice you can overcome all the negative programming you have done over the years so that you gain control over your habits, your thoughts and your behaviours. It's almost like emptying a dustbin so full of rotten rubbish that it makes everything around it stink! Oh yes, you can make huge positive changes to your weight and your life!

IMPORTANT: If you are clinically depressed or suffer from epilepsy, consult your GP before using these powerful techniques.

DAYS 1 AND 2: LEARN SELF-INDUCED RELAXATION

There are so many myths about hypnosis and hypnotherapy. Many believe that somehow they are out of control or vulnerable during a session of hypnotherapy but the truth is: this is not a general anaesthetic. What the hypnotherapist actually does is facilitate a process whereby the client can relax and enjoy a pleasant, deeply relaxed state that alters their state of conscious awareness – a bit like not being totally awake or totally asleep. And of course with guidance you will be able to do this for yourself so that you can begin a process of self-hypnosis. The first stage is to learn self-induced relaxation, a technique introduced by Michael Joseph, founder of the London College of Clinical Hypnosis. Using self-induced relaxation you can begin to access the 'Alpha' brainwave state, which is the key to starting to re-programme your mind. Mastering this will help you connect directly with your unconscious mind. So that you understand how important Alpha brainwaves are and what this all means, I will now tell you about the four distinct brainwave patterns all human beings experience:

- *Beta state:* When we are in a normal everyday state of awakening and engaged in mental activities, we are activating our 'Beta' brainwave state. The frequency of brainwaves in your Beta state is from 15 to 40 cycles a second. So, when you are concentrating on your work or engaged in conversation, you are in your Beta state (unless of course the person with whom you are talking to completely bores you!).
- *Alpha state:* Whereas Beta state represents arousal, 'Alpha' means the opposite: Alpha brainwave is slower and frequency ranges from 9 to 14 cycles per second. For example, once you have completed a task and decide to sit down and rest, it is likely you are in Alpha state. A gentle, relaxed walk in the garden or a daydream can also be representative of this brainwave state. Alpha is the

state a hypnotherapist will help you enter; it is also the one most helpful for communicating with your unconscious mind.

- *Theta state:* The 'Theta' brainwave state is slower than Alpha. Here, the frequency range is normally between 5 and 8 cycles per second. It is possible that someone experiencing hypnosis may drift so deep that they engage the Theta state. In Theta a flow of ideas may occur and tasks become so automatic that you are not even aware of them, such as walking into the kitchen and wondering why you have gone in there. It is a great state to access if you are trying to attain creative ideas or want a complete chill from life!

- *Delta state:* Here, the brainwaves are much slower and range from 1.5 to 4 cycles per second. Brainwaves never drop to 0 because that would indicate someone is brain dead. However, in a deep sleep it is quite common to experience 2 to 3 cycles per second. When you go to bed, you may read for a while before you go to sleep. Before putting the book down, it is likely you are in low Beta. As the book goes down and you turn off the lights, your brainwave will drop from Beta to Alpha. When you close your eyes and relax even further, your state drops to Theta and finally, as you fall asleep you enter Delta.

Now that you understand how your mind works and that the Alpha/Theta brainwave state is the one that best allows you to communicate with your unconscious mind you can begin practicing self-induced relaxation.

DAYS 3–5: OUT WITH THE OLD, IN WITH THE NEW

During Days 3 to 5, I want your mind to begin to understand that something is changing. For years you may have been used to eating too much high-fat, high-sugar junk food and eating your meals much too fast. Underpinning this was a belief that you would never lose weight and that weight loss was something that was difficult, hard work and you would always stay fat. We need your mind to begin to understand that the old negative habits are over for good and you are now changing and moving forward to a life of healthier eating patterns, as well as a belief that you can control your weight and enjoy the transition of mind, thought and actions that will drive you on to losing unnecessary fat. It's a little bit like the New Year routine when you open the door, wave 'goodbye' to the old you and say 'hello' to the new one. Of course you can do this consciously but I want your unconscious mind to be in harmony with your conscious logic. It is for this reason that for the next three days I want you to follow the protocol set out below. In doing so, make sure you find somewhere that is safe, warm and as free as possible from distraction; remember to turn your phone off, too. Avoid lying down as you may fall asleep. Instead sit upright in a comfortable seat with your hands gently placed on your thighs. Once this is done use the following steps to say goodbye to the old limiting beliefs and habits and say hello to more appropriate ones:

- *Step one:* Induce relaxation following the process explained earlier (see page 158).
- *Step two:* As you relax deeply, allow your mental

concentration to focus on the part that represents how you are right now when it comes to your eating habits, beliefs and feelings about weight loss. When I use the word 'part', I simply mean something that you can relate to, such as a word, colour, sound, a feeling or a combination of one or more. Take Natalie, with whom I recently worked. As she used this technique she told me the part representing her current state was a combination between the colour red and the word 'FAT'. She explained that it just came to her when she was deeply relaxed. This is quite a common occurrence because as you already know the unconscious mind will bring it to you without you really having to think.

- *Step three:* Once you have identified the part responsible for your current state allow your mind to go blank, then ask your unconscious mind to help you identify what you would like to replace it with. For Natalie this was a huge sign that read 'IN CONTROL AND SLIM'. She went on to explain that seeing the sign also made her feel excited and more confident that she would be slimming down soon and much more in control of her eating habits.

- *Step four:* Having identified the part responsible for your current state and the part that's about to become the new part, it's now time to mentally let go of the old and welcome in the new, more resourceful part that will help you lose weight and control it for the future. This cannot be simpler. As you relax deeply, engaging the Alpha or Theta state just let go of the old part on your out-breath and welcome in the new on the in-breath. As you breathe out, take your time and pay attention to what you see, hear and feel. Do the same as you breathe in. Continue for as many times as you feel appropriate. It's important to remember that as you do so your unconscious mind is beginning to understand that things are changing. Remember, it's out with old thought patterns and in with new ones.

- *Step five:* Finally, awaken yourself formally by mentally counting up from one to ten. Tell yourself that at the count of eight you will open your eyes and at the count of ten you will be fully wide awake, alert and every part of you will be back in the room, including the new part you have embedded into your mind.

Try to do this process twice a day and even more if you have the time.

DAYS 6–10: FOCUS THE MIND ON THE END RESULT

Visualisation is a powerful technique that will help you to make a lasting change to your weight and also motivates you forward. It is a great weight-loss tool and helps program your mind at the unconscious level to be what you want to be. The mental image you place in your unconscious mind of yourself as a slimmer person will help your body conform to that image. Once your mind is programmed with the proper mental image, it will start to work in assisting you to lose weight. As you visualise, let go of any remaining thoughts of past dieting that failed and instead see the slender body you want so that your unconscious mind can help make this become a reality. It will then begin to positively reinforce your body by aiding your eating habits.

Programming your mind into believing you can lose weight and visualising yourself at your ideal weight is extremely powerful. When you visualise seeing yourself as a slimmer person, this image will be transferred to your unconscious mind. And as you know, your unconscious is the driving force and nothing will beat it. If it's new to you, this process does take time to get used to, but bear with it and if you find it hard to visualise, just allow your mental concentration to focus on what it feels like to be slimmer or what you hear people saying about you as a slimmer person. If possible, mix all three states, although it's normal for one to be stronger. Many of my clients tend to have what is known as one dominant modality (i.e. they tend to see it, feel it or hear it), so don't get frustrated if you cannot visualise because you will definitely be able to take yourself into the zone of hearing or feeling yourself as a slimmer person.

So, for Days 6–10, focus your mind on the end result by:

- *Step one:* Engaging a state of self-induced relaxation, where and when it is safe to do so.
- *Step two:* Once you have deepened your state of relaxation, see, hear and feel the end result. If you see yourself slimmer, turn up the brightness of the colours and pay attention to what you are wearing and how you move now that you are slimmer. You may find that you can feel yourself slimmer. If so, increase the intensity of these

feelings: perhaps you feel confident, excited and proud. Or if you tend to hear the end result, then turn up the volume. Perhaps you can hear the compliments you are receiving and also your own inner voice telling yourself how fantastic you look now that you are slimmer.

- *Step three:* Spend about five minutes in this state allowing yourself to see, hear and feel what you are experiencing. Become really associated with the state as opposed to being dissociated. Get involved in what you see, hear and feel, and adjust your body language to match this state.

- *Step four:* Having spent time focusing your mind on the end result, begin now to count up from one to ten. At the count of eight, open your eyes and at the count of ten, tell yourself that you will be fully wide awake and every part of you will be back in the room feeling refreshed and rejuvenated.

Aim to carry out this technique twice a day and if you get the chance, try it at the end of the day in bed. Remember, this is you programming your mind for a positive result and that result is a slimmer, trimmer and more confident you.

DAYS 11–15: AFFIRM YOUR WEIGHT CONTROL

For the next five days I want you to mentally focus on sending a strong, direct suggestion to your unconscious mind that you are now firmly in control of your weight. I emphasise the word 'control' because this will help you lose weight *and* keep it off. Your affirmations will embed the command of control to help you manage your eating habits and avoid junk foods and binge eating. This process could not be simpler, just follow the steps below:

- *Step one:* Drift into a deep state of relaxation.
- *Step two:* Once you are completely relaxed, mentally focus on your first affirmation. This can be as simple as 'I am now in control of my eating habits' or 'I am in control of my portions and proud to eat less'. Remember to keep your affirmations positive so instead of suggesting 'I am not going to eat chocolate' say, 'I am free from chocolate and now enjoy more healthy foods'.
- *Step three:* In deep relaxation embed these affirmations for around five minutes. As you say them to yourself, you can even see the words or turn up the volume as you say them, as well as intensifying the feelings you have.
- *Step four:* After about five minutes awaken yourself formally by telling yourself that you will count up from one to ten and at the count of eight will open your eyes. At the count of ten, you'll be wide-awake and any feelings of numbness completely gone.
- *Step five:* Complete the process by having a good stretch, secure in the knowledge that you are now in control of your weight.

DAYS 16–21: PUT IT ALL TOGETHER

During your final week of this mind programming protocol I want you to put it all together so that you have a powerful combination of techniques using the immense power of your brain. This is key to letting go of old habits and adopting new positive ones that get you firmly on the path to sustainable weight loss. You will see, hear and feel yourself slimmer and finally, affirm that it's you who is in charge of your weight, not the unconscious memories and attitude that encouraged you to over-eat. Of course, you can continue to follow this process after 21 days to help improve your progress, motivation and positive attitude to weight loss and weight control. Use the following steps:

- *Step one:* Drift into relaxation and go as deep as possible so that you engage the Alpha/Theta state (see page 160-161).
- *Step two:* As you drift deeply, breathe out the old and breathe in the new for a few minutes. Once you have done so, allow your mind to go blank for a few moments before visualising yourself at a perfect weight. If you cannot see it, then hear it, or feel what it is like to be your ideal weight. Do this for a few minutes before finally affirming that you are now in control of your weight.
- *Step three:* Before waking yourself up using the normal procedure I have outlined again in the next step, mentally send other positive suggestions into your mind such as 'I'm proud of myself as I am now losing and controlling my weight' or 'I feel excited and confident moving forward'.
- *Step four:* Awaken yourself in the standard way by counting up from one to ten, opening your eyes at the count of eight, and then become fully awake at ten.
- *Step five:* Finally, take a good stretch, smile and feel proud of yourself for programming your

mind to be the slimmer person you want and deserve to be.

OVERCOMING A FOOD PHOBIA

There are many people out there who have aversions to certain foods but sadly this tends not to be crisps, cakes and biscuits but more often things like salad ingredients or a dairy-based product, such as yoghurt. If you have a phobia for certain healthy foods, there are solutions. A food phobia can affect day-to-day living and those with such phobias often report an overwhelming surge of emotion when they come into contact with certain foods. The sheer panic the food phobic experiences can be embarrassing, which in itself intensifies the anxiety.

The phobia is often developed after a bad experience where the food was present during a negative situation and to reverse the phobia by analysing its origins can be challenging. Also, we have to remember it can be as simple as being forced to eat all the vegetables on your plate when younger to the point where you felt sick. The good news is that to reprogram your mind, you don't have to spend hours analysing where the phobia comes from, instead follow some of the simple techniques below that I will highlight for you.

Over the years, treating many different clients, I have used hypnotherapy as a successful tool in supporting those individuals with food phobias. Hypnotherapy helps people to change the way that they think about the problem and programs their reaction to the problem for the better. Take Susan, for example, a 52-year-old with a phobia of fruit, who came to see me to explain that not being able to eat fruit was destabilising her weight loss and her health.

Susan explained that she hadn't eaten fruit since she was a child but recognised that as the years were passing, she should start eating it because of its nutritional value. We agreed to conduct three sessions of hypnotherapy in which I delivered a mixture of direct messages to her mind that the fear of fruit was becoming less strong, as well as utilising a number of creative mind programming tools to override the negative connotations around fruit.

We agreed to eat fruit together at the end of the third session and I assured Susan that I would face the phobia with her. Susan not only ate fruit that day, but she went to the supermarket to buy a trolley load! If you have a phobia of certain foods that you want to start eating, consider some of the practical things you can do to counter this, including:

- Try gradual exposure: Ask a friend to slice a small piece of the food in front of you. Allow yourself to sit comfortably looking at it until the anxiety subsides. It is impossible to remain anxious forever, so give it time. Once the anxiety has dropped, put a larger slice of the food on the plate.
- When you put a piece of the food in your mouth, mentally sing a nursery rhyme loudly! This is a distraction technique that will help to sufficiently confuse the mind as you eat.
- As you see the food in front of you, deliberately change your physiology. Sit tall and make yourself smile. It's impossible to feel terror at the same time as smiling! This will help reduce your anxiety and feelings about the food.
- Face your food phobia with a supportive friend and inside your mind visualise the end result of

being successful. Imagine how good you will feel once the phobia is conquered! Allow that clear outcome to be embedded deep in your mind.

• If your food phobia causes you to gag severely, always work with someone who is professionally qualified and experienced in working with those suffering from food phobias in conjunction with your GP's advice.

Linda's story

Linda is one of the warmest people I have ever had come to visit me. She was friendly, co-operative and desperate to lose weight and build up her confidence. On the outside, she would appear okay, but inside she was hurt. As I chatted with Linda I suggested we follow my standard three-session programme of hypnotherapy to help condition her mind to that of someone who is in control of their weight, as well as agreeing a number of practical motivational tools and the 80–20 meal plan (see also page 67). Linda agreed to my proposal and we set to work.

In session one, we set the clear goal. I asked Linda to describe in detail what she could see, hear and feel as the end result. Linda told me that she could see herself 25 kilos (4 stone) lighter and wearing jeans, boots and a tighter black top. She explained that she felt more confident and that she was walking with her head held high, as opposed to looking down at the floor. Then she added that she was looking more flirtatious and it felt good! Having described the end goal to me, I conducted a session of hypnotherapy helping her to create a focused concentration on the end result. After the session we agreed a number of motivational tools she could implement, such as buying a new outfit and carrying her fat picture around with her to remind her what a life of fat really meant. I also taught Linda self-hypnosis and asked her to practice this for the following seven days.

At the second session, I asked Linda to think through all of the activities she was undertaking to achieve her end goal. Among other things, she explained that she was eating better, walking with more confidence, being proud of becoming slimmer, flirting a lot more and leaving food on her plate. Once she had identified all these activities, I conducted a session of hypnotherapy to help embed them deep into her unconscious mind.

Homework from session two included developing her own 80–20 meal plans and using self-hypnosis to embed the activities deep into her unconscious mind so that they became new habits. At the final session Linda had already lost 5 kilos (10lb) and was smiling lots. Not only that but she looked younger, fresher and much more positive. This was a woman who had taken the process seriously, accepted personal responsibility and worked with me in programming herself for the better.

At the final session we reviewed the meal plans moving forward and agreed on further motivational strategies, including a swimsuit moment. Yes, at last Linda was ready to work towards getting into a bikini! It had been over ten years since she had dared to try it on, but the time felt right. Linda agreed to hang the bikini up in the house where she would see it daily. This would serve as a motivator, and one she relished.

I conducted the final session of hypnotherapy with Linda and from that day on, she has moved forward and is more in control of food, more positive and much more naturally conditioned to eat better and control her weight. And YES, she got into that bikini!

CONSIDER THE VIRTUAL GASTRIC BAND

Operations to shrink the tummy are featured more and more in the news these days, but for me the risk and expense of these surgical procedures is far too high. Obesity makes any surgery risky, anaesthetics become more difficult to administer and regulate, while additional health complications such as diabetes and high blood pressure only add to the increased risk from any surgery. As well as the arguments around surgical safety, there's the psychological impact of these operations, too. The number of people who have had stomach surgery over the last ten years has surged and of course, while I appreciate for some there can be no alternative, for the majority this is not the case.

Many operations fail because of the underlying psychological problems of the patient, including what led them to gain so much weight in the first place. Professionals recognise the huge potential for difficulties given the psychological problems suffered by patients and many agree it is those patients who should not be considered for such types of surgery. And there have been deaths following stomach surgery, including Suzanne Murphy (121 kilos/19 stone), who died after stomach stapling. For me the risks outweigh the benefits and it's the psychological risks that concern me as much as the surgical ones. If someone is eating because something is going on inside their mind, having surgery on their stomach won't solve this.

Some reports highlight a problem known as 'soft-calorie syndrome', where patients cheat by liquidising food. Some colleagues have told me tales of patients liquidising fish, chips, burgers and even chocolate bars! In America psychologists have found that some patients become alcoholics and even sex addicts after surgery, a condition known as 'addiction transfer'. This is because people often put their problems down to being overweight when in fact they are compulsive eaters and once the eating stops, another compulsion develops to replace the fixation on food.

After surgery, it is also possible that the patient is unable to eat as they used to and they may suffer anxiety and depression. Depression can deepen as the body image isn't what was expected and the sight of loose skin may shock. Of course, that's not to say there aren't exceptions out there, where this kind of surgery is of benefit. I guess my point is that often stomach surgery seems the easy solution but I am left questioning if cash-rich surgeons are telling us the whole truth about the success of this procedure.

Take the study of 317 gastric-band operations conducted

by Hôpital du Chablais in Switzerland in 2006, which at the time of writing found that after seven years fewer than half the operations could be deemed a success. This organisation also identified there can be problems with the device itself in that the band may start to migrate and lead to pain and irritation. Slippage, erosion and leakage are also potential problems, which can cause complications such as internal bleeding or infection. In the study of 317 gastric band cases conducted by M. Suter in Switzerland, an astonishing 33 per cent of patients developed late complications. Within this, 9.5 per cent of cases reported problems relating to the device itself, including band erosion.

Anita's story

As I continue to support people in their quest to lose weight I am often contacted by members of the public who share their stories of gastric band surgery disasters. Take Anita, who contacted me recently. She had heard an advertisement on local radio for a free seminar to understand more about gastric band surgery. Anita had been thinking about having a gastric band for a while and so she decided to go along and find out a little more about them. She had heard how many like herself had lost stones, even halved their bodyweight by having a gastric band, so after speaking to her husband (and with his support), she decided to go for it. She attended her first consultation and was shown 'before' and 'after' pictures of what to expect once she lived life with the band. With her current weight at 155 kilos (24 stone and 6 pounds) and a BMI of 55, she was eager to crack on.

Advised that she needed to lose a bit of weight before surgery, four weeks later Anita paid her non-refundable deposit of £1,000 with the balance due to be paid on the day of the operation. She was happy in the knowledge that she had a date for surgery and fully understood that in order for the operation to go ahead, she needed to get her BMI under 50 to make surgery safe. Anita told me that having spoken to other people she was made aware that before they had their surgeries they were evaluated by a psychiatrist to assess their mental health.

On the day of the operation Anita paid the outstanding balance of £6,000 to have the band fitted. Her band came with 12 months aftercare, too – which of course she was grateful for. She stayed at the hospital overnight and went home the next day. For the first four weeks after having the band, Anita was put on liquids and then moved onto other foods, such as mashed potato and gravy or custard for a further four weeks. Following this, she went onto normal food. Anita complained that following her surgery no one had contacted her to see how things were progressing, so after six months she complained and she was eventually given a refund for the aftercare of £1,000.

Anita explained to me that she had struggled since day one with the gastric band. Being able to eat smaller amounts of food meant that if she ate a little too much, it would make her sick and that having a band doesn't stop you eating foods such as cakes, biscuits and crisps because these are processed foods that go down easily. Anita did lose some weight, but even with a band she is now putting the weight back on. She now hopes to get a bypass on the NHS, but acknowledges that she needs to 'sort out her head' when it comes to overeating; she feels that if she doesn't do this first, no amount of surgery will help her shed the weight. Anita explained to me in her email that she feels like a time bomb ready to explode and that her family will be going to her funeral sooner rather than later. At just 53, she realises that her time on earth is limited if she fails to lose the weight. Anita told me that she would consider techniques such as Neuro-Linguistic Programming (NLP) to understand why she overeats and to help begin to turn her back on a life of fat.

Reading Anita's story made me realise that weight loss really is weight *control* and that it all starts in the mind. If the mind isn't focused, motivated and programmed in a way that is appropriate, no matter how much surgery people receive the problem will always be there.

THE HYPNOTIC ALTERNATIVE

You already know that I have a confidence in hypnotherapy, which lead me to train in using it to help people lose weight, and I am happy to report that the virtual gastric band is becoming increasingly popular with my weight-loss clients as its validity and reliability becomes internationally recognised. In simple terms, the virtual gastric band mimics surgical intervention as closely as possible without the need for an invasive and potentially dangerous procedure. It convinces the person using hypnotherapy that they have in fact undergone a clinical intervention. There are many forms of the virtual gastric band practiced in the UK, but all of them at some point closely model the real surgical procedure and work on the assumption that if we can imagine doing something, we can see ourselves doing and experiencing something, it increases the likelihood that we will in very real terms be able to do it. This is because the idea and the program for doing it have been stored in our memory just as if it were a real event and this is especially the case if the real issues that stop us from achieving are acknowledged.

So, what happens? There are many types of virtual gastric bands out there, however my own comprises four sessions, with two follow-up sessions as directed by the client. I developed my own protocol with Michelle Hague of the London College of Clinical Hypnosis. The process is structured to help condition the unconscious mind to think that the client has had a gastric band fitted, enabling them to eat less food so weight control takes place. Below I set out my own process in detail:

- **The first session:** During the first appointment a full case history is taken to find out about the client's weight-loss goals. I also explain the process in detail. At this session, body mass index is calculated and a 'before' picture taken. I am always keen to explain that the Steve Miller Virtual Gastric Band process is not a quick fix and will require homework, hard work and motivation on the client's part. The process includes assessing motivation, so clients are asked to complete an inventory, which helps to understand how motivated they are to this particular approach. If the motivation is not aligned to the virtual gastric band then other options are discussed.

  Oh yes, any hypnotherapist who guarantees an instant result is in my opinion acting dangerously and should be treated with suspicion – it goes against all the established professional ethics and regulations. A general session of hypnotherapy is facilitated so that the client begins to understand how hypnotherapy works. In addition, a strong rapport is created to move forward and enable the client to focus on the weight-loss goal.

- **The second session:** In session two, clients receive a structured nutrition plan using the 80–20 approach. This contains lots of foods that are raw and natural, fresh and simple, pretty plain and in small amounts. Nothing should be banned or excluded but refined and highly processed food that is high in sugars, salt and fats should be regulated and reduced. Unhealthy core beliefs and behaviours are identified and help is given to understand what is eaten, where it is eaten, when and why, and what unhealthy negative emotions are involved. This information helps to address bad habits and create new behaviours; also to confront emotional eating and identify practical strategies that can also be worked on using hypnotherapy. Procrastination is also something that needs to be looked at closely in the early discussions as it is often missed.

Dr Piers Steel, leading expert in motivation and procrastination, found in a long-term study that 42.2 per cent of people studied avoided or procrastinated about issues around diet and exercise. Goal setting is therefore imperative! Hypnotherapy in this session sets up the goal and commitment of the client to the procedure and the changes they will be making for the future. Visualisation is used to reinforce the ideas and goals that have already been discussed. Clients are asked to keep food diaries and to practice their self-hypnosis, which they have already been taught in session one. This is an important and necessary part of the process.

• The third session: In the third session, the client's motivation is checked and their commitment to change noted. If at this point the client is not displaying the right motivation then the process is suspended. Clients may decide to take a pro-rata refund or take time out to assess their motivation. If they are ready to go, the surgical procedure is discussed and to get the client further into the zone, they may wish to watch videos of the surgical procedure. The hypnotherapy in the third session is supportive of the surgical procedure to come: it carries with it the commitments and direct suggestions needed to help prepare the client and also gives the opportunity to reinforce the reality of what they are about to undertake and enhances its significance. Pre- and post-operative advice is given, the client will be advised not to eat prior to surgery and told that it is advisable to have someone to drive them home, to avoid heavy lifting and just to be mindful in the following few days. After all, the client is committing to have a virtual surgical procedure that must be made as realistic as possible.

- **The fourth session:** At long last the event that has been so carefully planned for and anticipated has arrived and in this, the fourth session, we carry out the surgical procedure. By this stage it is very common for the client to have already lost weight. The environment is carefully set for this session to help stimulate the client's senses, thereby helping to reinforce the emotional element of the experience. This may include sounds of the hospital or operating room, sensory stimulation such as the touch of a cotton-wool ball on the back of the hand as it is swabbed and smells, such as disinfectant.

  Once the session is complete aftercare is discussed and homework encouraged. A date and time for a fifth session is booked in for the band to be checked and for any possible adjustment needed. Of course, it may not need adjusting but it is better to have it checked to ensure maintenance. Adjustment to the band is a simple session, where checks on weight loss and statistics from the start can be made to review progress and behavioural changes. Any adjustments are made in hypnotherapy.

- **The fifth and sixth session:** As explained above, a fifth session focuses on any changes to the band. In addition, I always offer clients a sixth session for continued support. The sixth session may be a six-month check up or just a simple booster of motivational hypnotherapy. It may be that the client's requests to use the sixth session for an adjustment of the band or to re-establish goals alongside further support and encouragement.

The changes using the Steve Miller Virtual Gastric Band are potentially life changing and can be life-long, but you should be aware that this procedure is not appropriate for all clients looking to use hypnotherapy to lose weight. Alternative methods are available and I often recommend clients to undertake a series of weight-loss hypnotherapy sessions as opposed to the virtual gastric band. This alternative approach frequently brings better results and is more cost-effective for clients. If you are interested in hypnotherapy for weight loss, further details may be found by visiting www.thestevemillerplan.com.

SELECTING A HYPNOTHERAPIST

If you would like to work with a hypnotherapist there are some important areas to explore. First, I would strongly recommend you work with someone who specialises in weight loss. If a hypnotherapist is trying to be all things to all people it is less likely they will bring the experience of understanding the physiological, psychological, motivational and emotional aspects of someone looking to lose weight. When you make contact with a hypnotherapist, ask what qualifications they have, explore their experience and if it doesn't feel right, they are not for you.

Sadly there are no mandatory qualifications to set up as a hypnotherapist so it is important that you understand what they have achieved academically to train in hypnotherapy. Once they have informed you as to where they have trained, do an Internet search for the institution. If it doesn't appear professional, move on and talk to other hypnotherapists. If the hypnotherapist you call is offering low fees, be very cautious: cheap often means they are desperate for clients. At the time of writing, a successful practitioner will charge £70 as a minimum per consultation.

As you talk to the hypnotherapist ask how many sessions will be needed. A rough guide is three to six sessions; any less and the work won't be completed and any more means they are more interested in your money. Ask if they are a member of a professional body such as the British Society of Clinical Hypnosis or the National Council for Hypnotherapy. If they don't belong to a reputable organisation, walk away.

Finally, and very important, is the inspiration they offer you. If the hypnotherapist does nothing to impress when you initially meet, it is important to explain that you feel it isn't right for you. There is nothing to be afraid of if you decide to do this: hypnotherapy is very much about the relationship you will have with your practitioner and if they don't initially inspire you, then it's less likely the process will help you lose weight and what's more, you will be wasting your money.

MAKE EXERCISE A PLEASURE

Some of you may be completely horrified by the thought of exercise and believe it or not, I do understand. For you, the idea of going to the gym is almost like asking you to walk on hot coals or go straight into a cage of lions. Well, the good news is that if you are one of those people who really cannot bear the gym then you don't have to! For one, I'm not really a gym buff myself: I prefer to exercise for pleasure, not pain. Does exercise need to hurt? Do you have to feel the burn? The answer is NO! To be frank, I'm not an advocate for making people go to boot camps, or exercise so intensely they feel their limbs are about to drop off or they're about to faint. But of course you need to get a lot more active and while this will help you lose weight, it also supports your general state of health.

The secret of exercising is to simply identify an activity

you enjoy doing in your free time and in this chapter I will guide you through the alternatives. Ideally, you will do around an hour of exercise each day to help get your body moving and encourage the calories to keep on burning, but in doing so it's essential you mix and match your chosen exercise so that it keeps you interested, fits into your busy lifestyle and most of all, so that you enjoy it! For many the pay-off will be relatively quick and the weight loss sustainable because the body is burning up the healthy food you have adopted and the occasional '20' treat from the 80–20 rule. At the same time, it also uses up the stored fat you have accumulated.

Remember if you are new to exercise, returning to exercise or overweight check with your GP that it is safe to partake in the exercise of your choice.

THE BENEFITS OF EXERCISE

There are so many advantages to exercise, some of which you may not have considered. Let's take a look at them here:

- **Confidence is increased:** Increasing the amount you exercise is a brilliant way to increase your confidence and self-esteem, too. As you begin to look much better, you'll notice that you feel really good after a session of exercise as the endorphins (feel-good chemicals) kick in. What's more, the self-discipline gained from doing set exercise will have a positive effect on other areas of your life, at home and at work. Indeed, it can encourage your mind to become more orderly and open

to planning and setting routines for healthy
eating, food shopping, meal plans, playing with
the kids, etc.

- **The risk of heart attack is reduced:** Exercising definitely
reduces your risk of having a heart attack and
supports a lowering of cholesterol and blood
pressure.

- **Exercise helps with Type 2 diabetes:** If you suffer Type 2
diabetes, exercise can help reduce the impact it has
on your health and if you don't, exercise certainly
helps in the prevention of this condition, which
affects so many people because of poor lifestyle
choices.

- **Mental focus is increased:** Research shows that regular
exercise helps to keep the brain sharp as we get
older and impressively supports mental
concentration. Taking exercise also helps to reduce
your chances of developing Alzheimer's Disease.

- **Depression and anxienty are lessened:** The release of
endorphins through exercise significantly helps if
you suffer from depression and anxiety, as well as
improving your mood.

- **Posture is improved:** See your posture improve
naturally as you begin to exercise more frequently.
You will soon notice that you walk tall, holding
your head up high, and have greater presence
around people.

- **The risk of breast cancer is lowered:** Something that I found interesting is that estradiol and progesterone, two ovarian hormones linked to breast cancer tumour production, are lowered through exercise.

- **Stress is melted, as well as the fat:** Exercise really helps to melt away the stresses of life. If you find being stuck in traffic, conflicts with people, work and other everyday challenging situations stressful, build in some exercise after work. And *yes*, as your exercise levels increase and your stress levels decrease, your sex life will improve!

- **Exercise is benefical to the heart:** As you exercise more and more, your cardiac output increases, as does the contractility of the heart's ventricles. But the benefits don't stop there: the power, weight and size of the heart increases. That weight increase is fine, by the way!

So, exercise offers a range of benefits, both physically and mentally. But what exercise will suit you? Below, I offer my own views and ideas on a range of interventions to consider building into your lifestyle. Choose a couple of activities to avoid getting bored doing the same thing. Remember, this is not about making you into an Olympic athlete or muscle building champion – far from it! What I want you to do is simply to become more active in a pleasurable way to help you slim down and feel more confident.

WALKING

Not only is walking easy and straightforward, it's also free! Walking is my personal favourite exercise and brings many benefits including strengthening of the heart reducing stress and anxiety. Researchers have found that walking supports better thinking ability and helps build a clear focus on life. Even more importantly, research also suggests regular walking can help reduce your chances of breast and colon cancer.

There are a few types of walking. The first requires no technique at all in that you just go out and walk, putting one foot in front of the other. Let's face it, unless you have a disability, there's no excuse! As a nation, we have become extremely lazy and seeing people get into their cars and drive 200 yards to the newsagent does nothing to help reduce obesity levels. This, in my opinion, is downright laziness! Another type of walking, known as 'power walking', is also often referred to as 'speed walking' and all you need to do is increase the pace. In doing so, swing your arms forward and back, keeping them close to your body. To increase speed, speed up the swing of your arms and your legs will follow. If you haven't exercised in a long time build slowly up to a speed walking level. The ideal speed for walking is around 4.8–6.4km (3–4 miles) per hour, but if you are new to walking then a slower starting pace is fine. Why not buy a pedometer to calculate how many steps you have taken – they can be great as a motivational tool to help increase your walking coverage!

Walking doesn't need to be dull either. Make sure you plan and alternate a few routes and if friends or family want to join you, invite them along so you can have a natter en-route. Personally, I love walking with a dog so I often borrow my sister's dog to keep me company. Walking is superb for weight loss – take Stephen Fry, who lost 38 kilos (6 stone) in six months in 2009, using walking as his core exercise. You may also like to consider taking days out walking and if you prefer a flat terrain, try canal walking. Calorie burning using walking as your main form of exercise will of course depend on your current weight. However, a person weighing in at around 67 kilos (10½ stone) burns around 136 calories an hour with general flat walking. If you made that an uphill walk where more effort was required, he or she would burn around 400 calories. However, someone weighing around 127 kilos (20 stone) would burn around 554 calories an hour walking on flat terrain. As the effort and speed increases, so too does the calorie burn.

There are also some great websites to help you plan interesting walks, such as www.go4awalk.com, which is incredibly useful. If walking becomes your new hobby, you may even get brave and join the Ramblers Association. For information, visit www.ramblers.org.uk.

SWIMMING

Come on, where's your swimsuit hiding? Swimming is the perfect fun exercise to help you lose weight and what's more, it works all the muscles, helping you tone up at the same time. This isn't about making you into Tarzan, but about swimming at the local pool to burn off calories and melt the fat. What I love about swimming is that it's relaxing and playful and so many public baths now offer aqua-aerobic classes, making exercising in the pool brilliant fun and also very sociable. Swimming is a superb calorie-burning form of exercise and will certainly improve your heart's capabilities.

Because the whole body is moving when you swim your heart and lungs work hard to keep up the supply of oxygen, which means that swimming is a fabulous full workout. Exercise that makes you breathe harder is good because it shows your body is working overtime, which over time, will help to reduce your blood pressure. What I really love about swimming, though, is that because it's a great aerobic exercise, it really tones you up and as the whole body moves, it also helps to improve the flexibility of your muscles and joints. If you are sitting there thinking you'd love to take up swimming but are too embarrassed about putting on your swimming costume or your trunks, don't worry! First of all, you won't be the only overweight person at the pool and second, people at the swimming baths are much more focused on having fun and doing exercise than what other people look like. Do check out your local pool – many will have separate sessions for men and woman and also adult-only time, with lane swimming. Many also offer great aqua aerobics classes. They are fun and you can listen to music in the pool, which makes exercise more pleasurable! Remember, if you haven't swum for a while ask for advice on how to do a few exercises out of the pool before getting in.

One of the trends in recent years has been for people to swim in local rivers or ponds and in the sea. If you are lucky enough to live in a place where this is a possibility, go for it! Check online to see if there is a local club nearby that will guide you and get you into this free and stimulating exercise. Now I don't expect you to turn into David Walliams and swim 225km (140 miles) of the

Thames, but if you start off gently and go where that takes you, you'll lose loads of weight on the way. A word of warning: open water swimming can be dangerous so be cautious, and please don't swim in polluted water and rivers – you don't want to get ill. For more information about outdoor swimming visit www.wildswimming.co.uk.

In terms of calorie burning through swimming, listed below are some examples:

- Someone weighing 76 kilos (12 stone) burns around 231 calories every half hour of moderate swimming.
- A person weighing 95 kilos (15 stone) burns around 289 calories every half hour of moderate swimming.
- Anyone weighing 114 kilos (18 stone) burns around 347 calories every half hour of moderate swimming.
- A person weighing 140 kilos (22 stone) burns around 425 calories every half hour of moderate swimming.
- And finally, someone weighing 190.5 kilos (30 stone) burns around 579 calories every half hour of moderate swimming.

ZUMBA

If you fancy getting involved in the latest craze, maybe Zumba is for you. This Latin-inspired dance fitness class combines different dance styles together with aerobic exercise. It's a great way to exercise as it doesn't feel like you're working out as you're having so much fun! Zumba is also easy to follow and that's why it's so appealing to so many. If you really fancy taking up a new way to keep fit, but are nervous because you are overweight then don't be. As Zumba expert Mel Carpenter explains: 'All sizes, all shapes, all nationalities, all ages attend.' In fact, Zumba Basics is suitable for anyone aged 13 and over.

Zumba appeals to the masses because it's not your stereotypical aerobics class and is therefore not at all intimidating, especially for those new to exercise or returning after a break. It's excellent for weight loss, too. Take Mel, who went back to teaching Zumba just 15 weeks after giving birth and soon noticed she dropped *two* dress sizes! Calorie-wise you can expect to burn between 500 and 700 calories per session. If you would like to find out more about Zumba, visit www.zumba-central.com.

AEROBICS

Going to an aerobics class can be real fun for the many people who love working out to music. I remember attending a few classes myself and there was nothing better than exercising to some good tunes. Aerobic exercise is a cardiovascular exercise that is great for the large muscle groups. It makes the lungs work harder because the body needs more oxygen and helps to improve energy levels; it's also the perfect stress buster, helps lower your blood pressure and reduces the risk of a stroke or heart attack.

If you prefer not to attend a class then there's nothing stopping you from doing some aerobic exercise at home. All you have to do is put on your favourite CD and dance about the house but remember, it's aerobic and so the intensity should be high. If it floats your boat you can also take a look at buying some fitness DVD's or a Wii Fit (which is great for the family) to use at home, but be sure you are going to use them because they can be expensive.

Aerobic exercise is a great calorie burner as you lose weight, but remember to check with your doctor first that it is safe for you to do it. Typical calorie-burning results can be as follows:

- Someone weighing 76 kilos (12 stone) will burn around 222 calories every half hour of low-impact aerobics.
- A person weighing 95 kilos (15 stone) burns around 277 calories every half hour of low-impact aerobics.
- Anyone weighing 114 kilos (18 stone) burns around 333 calories every half hour of low-impact aerobics
- A person weighing 140 kilos (22 stone) burns around 407 calories every half hour of low-impact aerobics.
- And finally, a person weighing 190.5 kilos (30 stone) burns around 554 calories every half hour of low-impact aerobics.

JOGGING

If you want to turn walking into jogging, do so with care! Make sure you have checked with your GP first because this really is taking your exercise to the next level. Without doubt, jogging is a good way to improve your fitness levels and it's a great fat-burner, however you don't have to do it to lose weight and be fit. There is a myth out there that says running or jogging is the be all and end all when it comes to fitness. But I think that's nonsense! Good brisk walking does the same job, but of course if you really want to up the tempo, go for it with care.

Personal safety is important if you want to start jogging. Before you begin, make sure you have invested in some bright clothes to wear so you can be easily spotted, especially in the dark. It is also imperative that you invest in a pair of good-quality running shoes and start off with short distances because there is always the risk of long-term damage to the joints – it's all about being sensible. And a word of warning: when you do start running, be careful if you jog wearing earphones because it can be dangerous if you can't hear oncoming traffic.

When safety is assured there's no doubt that jogging makes the heart stronger and increases the capacity of blood circulation, too. Jogging also helps speed up the digestive system and improves respiration. In addition, you'll find it clears the head rapidly and endorphins are immediately released.

Jogging burns fat more quickly than any other form of exercise and certainly increases the metabolism, quickly burning off hundred of calories. If it's safe for you to start jogging, always do some stretches before each jogging session. These may include touching your toes or bending at the waist from side to side; remember to stretch your calf muscles, too (repeat at the end of your run). Start off at a gentle pace until you have warmed up. Following this, slowly build up the pace to a comfortable speed and before long you will work out what speed works best for you. I have talked with many people who have taken up jogging and they explain that their energy levels build up quickly and it's not long before they can extend the length of their routes, start running up hills, doing small organised runs, etc.

When you are coming to the end of your run slow down gradually and walk the last part of the route as this will help prevent the build-up of lactic acid in your muscles (if this happens, the muscles can get very stiff and uncomfortable). At this intensity I would advise you to seek guidance from an accredited personal trainer or a fitness instructor.

Jogging certainly burns the calories. Typically, you can expect the following:

- Someone weighing 76 kilos (12 stone) will burn around 267 calories every half hour of jogging.
- A person weighing 95 kilos (15 stone) burns around 333 calories every half hour of jogging
- Anyone weighing 114 kilos (18 stone) burns around 400 calories every half hour of jogging.
- A person weighing 140 kilos (22 stone) burns around 489 calories every half hour of jogging.
- And finally, someone weighing 190.5 kilos (30 stone) burns around 667 calories every half hour of jogging.

HORSE RIDING

For me, this is one of the most enjoyable forms of exercise. Not only does this sport work all the muscles, it also allows you to work with one of the most interesting animals on the planet! If you are keen to ride, then always consult a reputable riding establishment that runs their business aligned to strict health and safety regulations. Horse riding is particularly good once you have lost a decent amount of weight because unlike other forms of exercise, it isn't one that will burn the calories as quickly as some of those mentioned above but believe me, it does help!

The energy used to maintain a good posture and work with the horse helps burn fat and therefore reduces weight. What's more, it will also tone your muscles. Take a look at anyone who rides regularly – it's not often that you get fat on horseback! As you ride the horse, you will use your postural muscles as well as those in your arms and legs. In fact, you'll be working lots of muscles at the same time, which helps you burn calories and fat. Personally, I find horse riding good for posture because it develops the muscles symmetrically and weight loss tends to be around the middle and the thighs as these muscle groups get worked hard. Calorie-burning wise, expect the following per hour:

- Someone weighing 76 kilos (12 stone) will burn around 191 calories per hour of horse riding (walking).
- Anyone weighing 95 kilos (15 stone) burns around 239 calories per hour of horse riding (walking).
- And finally, person weighing 114 kilos (18 stone) burns around 287 calories per hour of horse riding (walking).

If you are above this weight, it is unlikely that you will be able to take up horse riding as a form of exercise until you have shed some pounds due to the safety of the horse.

SALSA DANCING

Oh, it looks *so* sexy and it's so much fun! Salsa is an expressive form of dance and an excellent way to burn around 10 calories per minute – it doesn't take long to pick the steps up, either. It's great to do if you have a partner, but lots of singletons go along, too. I've found it the perfect confidence-booster. The Salsa is an Afro-Caribbean dance and you'll enjoy learning twists, turns and lots of other hip-shaking stuff that really melts the fat. Calorie-wise, expect to burn between 200–400 calories an hour. Most towns and cities now run classes, so do a web search for the one nearest you.

CYCLING

Ever thought about getting on your bike? Cycling can be a fun and pleasurable pastime and you'll take in a lot of fresh air and scenery, too. It's a good choice for the whole family. As well as being great fun, cycling offers a challenging workout and can burn lots of calories. The calories burn as your heart rate increases, but also your strength increase because cycling exercises the muscles in the legs. Cycling is particularly suited to those who cannot do high impact sports because of their joints and it's therefore a good alternative to running or racquet sports. So long as you're not thinking a slow-bicycle race, your heart and lungs get a great workout, too! If you do decide cycling is for you then my advice would be to get a helmet, make sure you have lights on your bike and use reflector bands – you can't be too careful!

In terms of calorie burning, if you cycle for leisure as opposed to speed then some typical values are as follows:

- Someone weighing 76 kilos (12 stone) will burn around 151 calories each half hour of cycling.
- A person weighing 95 kilos (15 stone) burns around 189 calories each half hour of cycling.
- Anyone weighing 114 kilos (18 stone) burns around 226 calories each half hour of cycling.
- A person weighing 140 kilos (22 stone) burn around 277 calories each half hour of cycling.
- And finally, someone weighing 190.5 kilos (30 stone) burns around 378 calories each half hour of cycling.

HOUSEWORK

If you really feel uncomfortable going out to exercise then you can always stay home and do some housework! As with all exercise, you really do have to put the effort in here, though. Standing to iron next week's clothes is unlikely to burn much fat. Good workouts include polishing hard, dancing about while you dust and having a good sweep inside and outside the house. While on the subject of outside exercise, you may also want to consider weeding the path and mowing the lawn. Typically, you can expect to burn off the following:

- Someone weighing 76 kilos (12 stone) will burn around 221 calories per hour doing housework
- A person weighing 95 kilos (15 stone) burns around 277 calories per hour doing housework.
- Anyone weighing 114 kilos (18 stone) burns around 332 calories per hour doing housework.
- A person weighing 140 kilos (22 stone) burns around 406 calories per hour doing housework.
- And finally, someone weighing 190.5 kilos (30

stone) burns around 554 calories per hour doing housework.

EXERCISE FOR THE DISABLED

For those of us fortunate enough to be able-bodied, exercise is fairly straightforward. However, for those disabled and in wheelchairs it can be more difficult. But you only have to watch the Paralympics to see and be inspired by the incredible and positive attitudes of people with disabilities, and their determination to exercise and take part in sport.

I feel passionately that people with disabilities should receive guidance on how to exercise, so I have taken it upon myself to do some research. It's essential for anyone in a wheelchair to keep the body moving as much as possible and this should become part of your daily routine. Regular wheelchair exercise will help increase strength, improve personal mobility, help ensure a healthy heart and lungs and of course if you need to lose weight, it will do just that. It's important to start off with a gentle warm-up, stretching a little without causing pain and discomfort, before taking ten minutes or so to cool down afterwards. Include exercises for the arms, torso, neck and shoulders.

I must stress that it is essential for anyone with a disability who wants to take up exercise to check this out with a doctor first to ensure it is safe to do so. It is vitally important to discuss what exercise is planned to and seek your GP's advice on what should be avoided.

There are two types of exercise for those in wheelchairs. The first is resistance training, where large rubber bands are used. These bands are wrapped around a secure object, such as a door or one arm of a wheelchair, before being pulled to give the muscles a good workout. The bands may be used for shoulder rotations and arm and leg extensions, too.

The second type of exercise is called strength training, where the disabled person uses weights or dumbbells. If no weights are available, it's fine to use cans of food. It is always advisable to start off with a light weight before moving on to something a little heavier. As with all exercise, it is important to seek advice from your GP before embarking on a new exercise regime. This will help to ensure that it is safe and appropriate.

For those of you who feel like you need extra incentive to exercise, it may also be worth consulting a qualified personal trainer for advice as many trainers are able to formulate bespoke plans taking into consideration a person's disability.

DO IT AS
A FAMILY

Perhaps your family needs to get slimmer, trimmer, fitter and healthier? If so, doing it together is a great way to melt the fat! Having worked with numerous families over the years I cannot say enough about how motivational this can be. Not only does it bring positive support but family members can be great at kicking each other up the backside to get on with it! In this chapter I want to share with you some of the practical strategies I have asked families to adopt to lose weight successfully. Use the ones that you believe will support your family best. If it is impractical to do it as a family then why not consider doing it with your flat-mate or a group of friends.

DEVELOP THE FAMILY MISSION

There's no better starting point than to sit down and agree on what you all want to achieve. Together, agree the end result in terms of what each member will weigh at the conclusion of the weight-loss journey. If you are involving the kids, make sure you have consulted a doctor, and if appropriate a dietician, to check that the plan is suitable for them. Once you've got the all-clear from the professionals, stress to the kids that this is about being sensible and getting fit and healthy and not looking like a stick-thin model in a magazine! If your kids are a healthy weight, then for them, this will be about getting healthier and, of course, supporting Mum and Dad! Take a large piece of colourful card and write down on it the words 'Mission Fit'. Add each family member's name and the aims each of you want to achieve, whether these are weight loss or fitness related. If you are in doubt as to your ideal weight, check with your GP first. Once you have done this, secure the mission on a wall where it will be seen daily. Now comes the fun part! Kids love to play so once you have placed the mission on the wall explain that you are going to agree as a family all the things you will do to help achieve that mission.

Hand out some smaller, bright colourful cards and agree one at a time what you are going to do to reach your goals. As you do so, make sure only one family member speaks at a time so everyone has his/her own airtime. It is always a good idea to sit at the table for this so that you have something solid to work on. Examples may include doing a family walk together every evening, eating three healthy meals a day using the 80–20 Plan (see page 67), or playing ping-pong together twice a week. Whatever is written down is what you sign up to so make sure the whole family buys into it before you write it down on the card. Once everyone has agreed what the actions will be on separate cards, place them on the wall around the mission. This forms the basis of your 'mission plan' – moving forward together as a family.

MEAL PLAN TOGETHER

At the beginning of each week plan together what meals you will eat as a family using the 80–20 rule, but then go one stage further and agree who will be cooking them. Try and share responsibilities and if you are cooking from recipes, involve the kids. The best education for living a healthy life that they can receive is definitely in the home, so encourage them to roll up their sleeves and help in the kitchen. It amazes me these days how many young adults can't even boil an egg, so involving the young ones helps massively. Furthermore, ask the kids to make the weekly shopping list with you so that they experience what a healthy weekly shop from the supermarket looks like.

MAKE IT EXCITING

For so many people, losing weight and becoming healthier starts off with all good intent but by week three, their motivation can quickly drop. The reason for this is because they become bored and lose focus on the end result. It is therefore crucial to make the whole journey as a family exciting. Consider building into your plan a number of rewards. These don't have to be big things; it can be as simple as going to the cinema together after a week of successful healthy eating and exercise or taking a trip to a theme park. Of course, it's always useful to include a bigger reward, such as agreeing that when the family has met certain goals you will all go to the travel agents and book a holiday. Another way to make it fun and exciting is to agree forfeits. Simply write down together a number of forfeits that could be done if a family member doesn't live up to what's been agreed each week and put them in a hat. If someone doesn't do what they said they were going to do, agree as a family if they deserve a forfeit. If they do, get them to pick one out of the hat! Forfeits could include having to clean the house for an hour, cut the grass or do the washing up for a week!

TAKE UP FAMILY HOBBIES

As you set out on Mission Fit it's a good idea to select a new family hobby or interest. There are several reasons for this. First, we pick at food when we become bored, so keeping busy really helps you forget about it. Second, many hobbies include activity and will burn off some calories as you do them and third, taking up a family hobby helps to bond and build family unity.

So, what kind of hobbies could you consider? Geocaching (www.geocaching.com) is something kids love! Using GPS navigation devices you set out to locate hidden pots of 'treasure' in a cache. It builds excitement and is such great exercise as you make your way as a family to find them. My sister and her family do this frequently and she says it gives them far more motivation to walk further than they would normally do. The use of the technology and the Internet helps find the locations and it can be great fun.

Inexpensive adventure days out are more widely available than you might think. The National Trust (www.nationaltrust.org.uk) is an independent charity offering lots of advice on places to visit as well as national events, such as walking festivals, wild child events and other great days out. At the time of writing, annual family membership costs just over a pound a week (children under five years old are free) and you will receive regular news and free car parking to most National Trust countryside, woodland and coastal car parks. In addition, you receive a member's handbook as well as three editions of the National Trust magazine. For further information, visit their website.

If you have the room, purchasing a table tennis kit is a great idea to boost the family's fun exercise. The good news is that playing table tennis is safe for all the family, it gets everyone running around, provides a great cardiovascular workout and it's also tons of fun! If you like the idea of this, setting up regular competitions is a good way of motivating all family members to get involved. Table tennis is also a good calorie-burner. For example, someone weighing 76 kilos (12 stone) can expect to burn around 151 calories if they play for one hour.

Picnic days out can be a real treat and another way to eat healthily as a family. Think about packing the car with some tennis rackets or Swingball, or if you have bikes perhaps take them with you. That way you can all enjoy time together burning some extra calories as well as enjoying a healthy meal. Here's a suggested picnic pack for your cool box:

- Large bowl of mixed salad.
- Lean ham and turkey slices.
- Low-fat mayonnaise.

- Wholemeal pitta breads – two each.
- Carrot sticks and low-fat hummus.
- Strawberries and mixed fruits.
- Low-fat yoghurt.
- Small chocolate bar (25g/1oz) each.
- Pure fruit juice, not 'juice drinks'

IF IT'S RIGHT FOR YOU, CONSIDER A DOG

For years my niece and nephew nagged my sister (who was 32 kilos/5 stone overweight at the time) to buy a dog. But she resisted, explaining that the time wasn't quite right and they would need to wait a few years. As the years passed the nags persisted until finally, she and her husband caved in and introduced Bobby, a West Highland terrier, into the family. At first, my eager niece and nephew enjoyed taking him out on long walks but as the novelty began to wear off, my sister (who was still overweight) decided to become the family dog walker.

As the weeks went on, she began to notice that the more exercise she gave the dog, the more she herself wanted to exercise. For years she had been chained to the house looking after the family, but Bobby actually got my sister's bum to move more and she loved it! Week after week she would walk miles and having blamed an under-active thyroid for her weight gain, she soon noticed that the more she moved, the more weight she lost. As she slimmed down, she realised that Bobby had become her walking machine and now several stone lighter, she enjoys a new lease of life and energy.

Of course, if you are tempted to buy a dog then it's important to think your decision through carefully. Dogs are not as independent as cats and they need so much more human attention and exercise. Here are the questions the Kennel Club (www.thekennelclub.org.uk) request you answer if you are thinking about having a dog as a pet:

- Can I afford to have a dog, taking into account not only the initial cost of purchasing the dog, but also the ongoing expenses, such as food, veterinary fees and canine insurance? As a very rough estimate, a dog can cost £25 [at the time of writing] a week.
- Can I make a lifelong commitment to a dog? A dog's average life span is 12 years.
- Is my home big enough to house a dog?
- Do I really want to exercise a dog every day?
- Will there be someone at home for a dog? Dogs get lonely just like humans.
- Will I find time to train, groom and generally care for a dog?
- Will I be able to answer YES to these questions every day of the year?

If you have answered 'no' to any of the above, you should think again before buying a dog.

PLAN TO MANAGE TEMPTATION TOGETHER

We are constantly faced with numerous social gatherings, such as weddings, birthday parties and family visits, which normally always include food and drink. When such occasions rear their head make a family pact that you will support each other. Agree a few actions you will take together, such as drinking low-calorie drinks and checking each other's portion control as you put food onto your plate.

Here, the key thing is that you give each other support.

Take a wedding, for example, where the buffet is stacked high and the alcohol is flowing fast. During the wedding have supportive chats with each other about how well each member of the family is doing and if anyone is struggling, agree to have a little pep talk. Of course there is nothing wrong with a couple of drinks, but if you fear this will lead to more it might be an idea for you all to go cold turkey on the day.

DRAW BODY SHAPES AS A FAMILY

Fancy some creative time? Consider getting together to draw your family's body shapes as they will be when the weight drops off. Once each of you has drawn your own shape, show it to each other. If you notice the kids are drawing body shapes that are too thin, discuss this with them and encourage them to draw their shapes again, which helps them to understand that too thin can be as bad as too fat.

Put the drawings on a wall or the fridge, where everyone will see them at meal times. This will help reinforce the end goal for all family members.

TAKE PICTURES OF EACH OTHER AS THE WEIGHT DROPS OFF

As the weeks pass, there's no doubt you will begin to see changes in one another's body shape. Consider taking photographs four weeks into your new lifestyle and posting these next to an original picture where you are certainly heavier. This can be a real motivator as you see the family change shape and look younger, fresher and healthier. If any member of the family has struggled, then leave the photograph and agree to take it next time. You might even consider starting a family photo album to illustrate the journey you are following together. This will be something to look back on with real pride when you all hit your ideal weight.

SECRET 12

ENJOY LOOKING GORGEOUS

You may think your body's not perfect, but I will tell you that having a positive body image is difficult to get and often we have a distorted view of ourselves. If you're not sure about the way you look and how others perceive you, then why not ask a trusted friend to give their honest opinion.

However, you have already purchased this book and begun taking steps towards a slimmer, healthier and happier you. So, when you reach your ideal weight, something I have full confidence in, what are you going to wear? Losing the initial pounds is no mean feat and in doing so, you will inevitably find yourself with nothing, or very little to wear. But fear not because help is at hand! I have consulted Luke Sutton, one of the UK's top image consultants and personal shoppers, and in this chapter, I share his tried-and-tested secrets from the image industry, which work well for people who are losing weight. Yes, it's time to talk glam!

FLATTER YOUR CURRENT WEIGHT, SHAPE AND SIZE

While losing weight, plan around your image because looking and feeling gorgeous will give you the motivation, confidence and enthusiasm required to achieve your final goal weight. This may seem pie in the sky, but believe me taking those small steps to show off your gradually reducing figure will help you and you'll also receive appreciation from those around you.

Image consultant Luke Sutton says that he has known women who try to plan their wardrobe around their distant weight-loss goal but when they cannot fit into the clothing they have bought and feel as though they have wasted hard-earned cash on beautiful clothing they simply cannot squeeze into, they are left feeling deflated and unmotivated. This of course allows their weight-loss programme to fall apart, they gain weight too easily and the goal is therefore lost. So, of course go out and buy items of clothing a little smaller but if you are currently a size 20, go for a size 16 initially as opposed to a 10. When it comes to your goal weight, just use a bit of common sense and work to sensible milestones that you can achieve along the way.

KEEP COSTS LOW

Most stores have a selection of discounted clothing tucked away somewhere. And for a style-savvy slimmer such as yourself this should be your first port of call when out shopping. Don't be afraid to ask retail staff where the bargains are because in the foreseeable future the clothing is not going to fit, so plan your wardrobe inexpensively around your current weight, shape and size. This allows you to update periodically at minimal cost, but gives you the right and opportunity to feel beautiful and enthusiastic throughout the duration of your weight loss.

WEARING BLACK IS A MYTH

Through his career as an image consultant and personal stylist Luke has come across some ridiculous style notions that need to be tossed out the window. A good example is the common assumption that wearing black is universally flattering when of course it's totally untrue that black suits everyone. For many women and men, more often than not those who are concerned about their weight shape and size, black is the easy option as they believe it looks good on everyone and is also slimming and complements all skin tones, eye and hair colours. In reality, black creates a merciless silhouette emphasising your outline, including all those lumps and bumps we despise. Also, when used in a block, black doesn't have the same disguising effect as carefully chosen colours, prints, fabrics and shapes used to draw the eye to the best areas and detract from those areas you are not so fond of. Having made this point, you must understand that bright colours can make you look larger but being plus-size doesn't mean you are doomed to a life of drab and unflattering outfits. Don't dismiss bright colours, simply learn to balance them with a darker colour that you know flatters your colouring.

A STITCH IN TIME SAVES NINE

Tailors and seamstresses provide a relatively cheap solution to perfecting your wardrobe, particularly for those with unusual proportions. It's surprising how dramatic the effect of a shortened sleeve or reduced hem can be. Simply changing the buttons or re-dying a garment may be all that's necessary to give it a new lease of life.

Alterations are not just for petite women whose clothing needs to be made smaller. Fuller-figured ladies and gents can add definition and shape to their body by using a tailor. I find that many individuals who consider themselves overweight and may suffer from low self-confidence as a result will wear loose-fitting clothing in an attempt to hide their figure from the world. Yet for women in particular this only delivers a blow to your curvy proportions as you go from the epitome of femininity to clothed catastrophe! No matter what adjustments you decide are necessary to revamp your style – whether shortening the length of trousers or completely obliterating every jacket you own – always invest in a tailor because they have the experience and knowledge of how to modify a garment and deliver the right result.

AIM FOR FITTED, NOT SKIN-TIGHT

On the opposite end of the scale from those who wear clothing that is too loose-fitting are the ones who squeeze into sausage-skin styles that are simply too tight. Stylist Luke Sutton has a frequent saying – 'skim, not skin' – that he finds works well when you are choosing garments for fit. Clothes should not be like a second skin, they should fit close enough to look good, but not reveal every bump and lump on your body.

DISCOVER YOUR REAL MEASUREMENTS

These days, tag sizes have little meaning since the actual sizes vary so much between designers, stores and brands.

Recognise that no matter how gorgeous or well made a garment might be, if it doesn't fit you properly then it will not look good. The only way to know for sure is to know your accurate measurements and head for the fitting room to try things on for size before you make a purchase. Do not rely on the measurements you took a few months ago, particularly while losing weight, as they will have changed. Knowing your real size is vital to getting a proper fit and so intimidating as it might feel, get out that tape measure and take those measurements all over again! Write them down so you remember and be sure to check your size at least every fortnight so you can shop for the right fit. For women, I would add that it is useful to get professionally measured for a bra regularly while you are losing weight as you can easily change your back or cup size as the weight drops, and what's more you will look even better as a well fitting bra flatters your whole figure as well as making the most out of your assets!

UNDERGARMENTS

By virtue of the name it will come as no surprise when I tell you that these garments are intended to go *under* your outer clothing, so keep your straps under wraps! Personally, I detest the sight of frilly knickers showing from beneath low-rise jeans or the bow detail on a bra poking out of an unbuttoned shirt collar. And yes, the sight of a white bra from beneath a dark coloured top and knitwear isn't that attractive! So, keep your bras and lacy panties out of sight... until you get an evening alone with your partner, of course. Cheeky!

The healthy way to walk in heels

As you shed the pounds week after week, you'll begin to envisage a slimmer, healthier and ultimately, happier you. For women especially this can be the visualisation of yourself blowing the dust off certain wardrobe treasures and getting back into chic flattering pieces: feminine frocks, sexy skirts and not forgetting those show-stopping stilettos!

The clatter of heels on the lobby floor might be somewhat of a distant memory and regrettably, so too could be your ability to walk in the darn things! But there is a solution: the secret to walking correctly in heels is to adopt good posture through knowing your centre of gravity. It is also important to feel confident in your heels and standing tall with your shoulders back and your head up not only improves the way you walk, but radiates confidence and authority to your peers. When you walk, pay attention to the palms of your hands. If they are facing backwards, you have bad posture so roll your shoulders back, stand tall and get comfortable with this stance. Ideally your palms should be facing inwards towards your body.

Still struggling? Imagine the clothes hanger has been left in the jacket you are wearing; also that this hanger is attached to your shoulders and someone much taller than you has taken hold of it and is now pulling tightly. So, what happens? Your shoulders go back, you pull your stomach in, your chest is pushed out and you stand tall. Did you notice how you took a deep breath in as you did this exercise as well? Now that's good posture!

TRY EVERYTHING ON

In an ideal world, everyone would try on clothing before making a purchase, but I've come to realise that few do and this is something I find completely mind-boggling! No one knows the intimate details of your figure better than yourself, so can you really be sure how a garment will look without trying it on first? Of course you can't, so head for the changing rooms at once, like any other style-savvy shopper!

THE FOLLY OF ONE MAN IS THE FORTUNE OF ANOTHER

Everyone loves a bargain and charity shops today offer quality clothing at rock bottom prices, as do many other thrift stores. If you fancy sifting through reams of clothing you may find yourself with some real treasures. However, it's important not to compromise on quality simply because of the price tag.

If delving into piles of clothing isn't your idea of fun and you have the Internet available to you, eBay can also be a great way to expand your wardrobe. Another source might be 'The UK's Online Marketplace' if you have a general idea of what you intend to buy and the time and patience. As I suggest elsewhere in this chapter there's no need to spend a fortune to look a million dollars but you should always opt for the best quality available within your budget. Once this clothing is too large for you and you have no further use for it other than to insulate your wardrobe, you may be able to recoup some of the costs by reselling various items through means such as eBay. Your average online bargain hunter knows a great deal when they see one, so invest your time wisely by selling the better-quality items at a price you know these deal-driven divas won't be able to resist.

Also, remember you can make a few extra pounds to invest in a new wardrobe for the slimmer you by selling your 'fat clothes' online. As you'll learn below, I want you to get rid of them as soon as you can. Naturally, there will be others out there who will appreciate your good taste and be eager to grab a bargain to fit their lardier bottoms into!

LOSE YOUR 'FAT WARDROBE'

Frankly, I find the notion of a 'fat wardrobe' versus a thin one infuriating. By holding on to your unwanted clothing you are tempting fate and making it all a little too easy for yourself to slip back into old habits. Aside from my advice to rid yourself of this clothing, that has previously left your confidence at an all-time low, there is little else to be said on the matter. So, de-clutter it now! Remember, it's out with the old and in with the new.

CHOOSE VERSATILE CLOTHING

To make full use of your wardrobe throughout your weight-loss journey, one golden nugget of advice that I would like to share with you is to think about the adaptability of every item you currently own and of those you are considering buying. Garments with high elastic content (particularly trousers) and the ability to shrink as you do are items worth considering. A top that may be very loose could work equally as well as a slightly looser or belted garment and again, this is a great option to add extra versatility to your wardrobe. For this principle to be effective takes a certain element of creativity and for you to have adapted a keen eye for style and understood the basic principles of your body shape and how to dress it. Without this knowledge experimental style can pose a real challenge so make sure you know what works for you!

EXPERIMENT AND HAVE FUN

Modern society places increasing focus on our appearance and what we wear presents a visual representation of the type of person we are. So, what do your clothes say about you? Of course it's essential when putting together a look that the rules of style are observed, but what's far more important is that we express some individuality and have fun experimenting with clothes, accessories and colour.

Keeping your style fresh and evolving maintains enthusiasm and confidence. Indeed, the confidence you display when you feel at ease in what you are wearing always shines through and will enhance any outfit.

INVEST IN AN IMAGE CONSULTANT

I'm the first to say that I am no style guru, however there are professionals out there who will do a good job in helping guide you to wear what is right for you. As a former fat boy I remember the fun I had improving my image and the confidence and motivation that gave me to keep on losing weight was huge. Typically, an image consultant will tell you your best colours, patterns, cuts, textures, styles, fabrics and prints. An *excellent* consultant, however, will go deeper than this and explore what truly makes you, *you*! To find out more, visit www.lukesutton.net.

PLAN TO KEEP IT OFF

So, once the weight has dropped, how do we keep it off? This is probably something that concerns you most and you are right to wonder how you will keep the slimmer shape that you now have. When you think about it you could probably name several people you know who have lost weight only to find months later, they have put it all back on. You already know that in my opinion restricted diets do not work and never will. While they are sometimes useful in getting the weight off, they rarely help people to maintain the weight long-term and that's why the 80–20 Plan is crucial from the start, helping you to learn to eat a little better while of course never denying yourself the occasional McDonald's breakfast or the KFC take-away.

Indeed, several studies reinforce my approach to long-term weight control. One study in the US found that people generally lost between 5 and 10 per cent of their weight during the first six months of dieting but shockingly, the review of 31 previous studies of weight loss found that within five years, up to two-thirds put more weight on than they had lost. Researchers also explain that losing weight and then putting it all back on also carries risks, among them heart disease and stroke, so not only does the restricted dieting philosophy affect people emotionally as they put it all back on, but it carries significant health risks, too. Researcher Traci Mann concluded from her studies that most people who lost a lot of weight and then put it all back on would in fact have been better not losing it at all, given the wear and tear on their bodies through losing it and then regaining it all.

In one study, a group of dieters weighed more than 6 kilos (11lb) over their starting weight five years after the diet (this didn't refer to one diet in particular, but took a broad spectrum). Now you can probably understand why I continue to fight against restriction in food plans! The secret is to have a range of strategies in place to help ensure the lifestyle remains healthy and conducive to long-term weight control. In this chapter I recommend my top three strategies to help you keep the weight off once you have lost it. Incorporate these into your lifestyle and you will maintain the healthy weight not today, not tomorrow, but for the rest of your life.

STRATEGY 1: EMBED THE NEW HABITS

By following my guidance in previous chapters you will continue to make significant progress towards your weight-loss goals. However, the secret is to consistently embed these new habits into your lifestyle, reminding yourself that if you let go of them then you will once again get fat – and possibly, even fatter. This may sound a little harsh, but it's true. Planning to embed the new habits will eventually mean your lifestyle is one aligned to long-term weight control, ensuring the fat never returns. Consider the following actions to help make sure your healthy habits are firmly in place. Use self-hypnosis twice a week to help keep your mind programmed on weight control (*see also* page 158). Remember, it's 'weight *control*' and not 'weight loss' at this point. Doing self-hypnosis helps keep the programme of weight control embedded in your unconscious mind.

You could write down what you do each week. This is different to a food diary in that you simply write down what you have achieved successfully in controlling your weight during the week and conversely what you will do moving forward to eliminate any bad habits that might have reared their heads. For example, simply writing down that you controlled your food well and how proud you felt at work when someone offered you a huge slice of birthday cake but you had a tiny piece. It could also include how you forced yourself out of bed a few mornings to do a one-hour brisk walk before getting ready for work. However, you can also write about anything that you will correct during the following week. For example, you could have been out a couple of times in the week and drank a little too much wine. Rather than beating yourself up about this, you may write about how you recognise that last week you drank a little too much and so to correct this, you have decided to go alcohol-free this coming week. That reminds me, I'm not suggesting you do this on a daily basis (unless you want to), but spend around half an hour each week jotting things down. This will help reinforce your new lifestyle and discipline you towards long-term weight control.

Alternatively, use positive affirmations daily. You already know how important it is to use positive self-talk (*see also* page 13). Now let's remember that every thought you think, every word you say is an affirmation of who you are. With the weight off, all your self-talk or inner dialogue associated with controlling your weight will be a stream of affirmations. In short, you will be affirming unconsciously with your words and thoughts and these will determine your results in moving forward.

Remember, your affirmations need to remain positive because negative affirmations about weight control will sabotage your efforts in achieving certain goals, in this case keeping the weight off long-term. What will also be important is your ability not to let others affirm for you. With the weight off, don't be surprised if you hear others saying, 'Oh go on, you've lost the weight now so another piece of cake won't hurt you' or 'Come on, don't be so boring! You've lost the weight, so another curry this week will be okay'. If you decide to accept what these demons say then you will be affirming to yourself that losing control is okay. So yes, listen to what they say so you don't appear rude but always decide if you want to accept what they tell you. Perhaps you're wondering what affirmations you can use to help keep the weight off. Here are a few ideas:

- Today I'm proud to be in control of my weight for good.
- For me, being in control of my weight is now natural and I do it with ease.

- Today I reinforce the control I have with food and the support it gives to my confidence.
- As I move forward I'm so excited, knowing I'm in control of my new, slimmer sexier shape.
- I love being in control of my weight as I live by healthy habits, following the 80–20 rule of eating.
- I'm proud of the thoughts I hold about my new slimmer shape and I know that others want a bit of what I have!

STRATEGY 2: BE FIRM AND MAINTAIN A LIFELONG AVERSION TO FAT

One of the best strategies in my book is to create a long-term aversion to being too fat but I must strongly point out that this isn't about crossing the thin line and being so anti-fat that you never eat the odd bit of 'junk' food again. Furthermore, in my book an obsession with fat is a complete no-no, so making sure the aversion is a healthy one is important. A healthy aversion means that you develop yourself to be naturally averse to unhealthy fat and what it does to you and other people.

To help create this aversion you have to maintain an awareness of yourself and others. You also need a mind that isn't focused on being politically correct and one that takes a dim view of excuses! Now the weight is off, if you dare to hear yourself making excuses for getting fatter, then immediately give yourself a good talking to. In your mind send yourself off to the headmaster's (or headmistress's) office for fat detention! Yes, tell yourself that excuses are forbidden and you are mentally writing five hundred lines that read 'excuses keep you fat, so I'm getting rid of them immediately'.

This may sound a little crazy but it is this lack of long-term discipline that allows those who have lost weight to pile it all back on again. Of course it's never a popular strategy, but it works well in giving you a short, sharp reality check. Once you have given yourself a dose of the truth, then tell yourself that the positive focus is back on and you won't be heading off to Fatsville city ever again. I am also a fan of keeping an old 'fat' picture of yourself close at hand so that if you are ever tempted to fall off the wagon you can remind yourself what life is like to be fatter. But creating an aversion to becoming fat again goes a little further than administering tough love to you for it involves others, too.

Now the weight is off, make sure that you continue to observe the negative habits of fat people. Notice what they eat, look at how fast they eat it, and study their shape closely. Then ask yourself: 'Is that how I want to look?' I also want you pay attention to their shopping habits. At the checkout, glance in a fat person's trolley and ask yourself the following question: 'Is it any wonder they are fat?' Observe fat people in public places doing their best to fit into the seats at the cinema, theatre or planes and notice how they struggle to stand for too long at a pop concert or a sports match. When on holiday notice how they fill up their plates and go back for thirds, never mind seconds, before spending the day lazing by the pool, allowing the calories to turn to fat. Remember, this is not about being cruel to people, it's the reality and of course the truth does hurt. Just imagine you being like them, and allow this image to deter you from copying their habits. Let this process reinforce your determination to stay slim, trim, more healthy and confident.

STRATEGY 3: EMBRACE THE 80–20 PLAN

The 80–20 Plan is straightforward, practical and a method of eating that you can use for life. Since it avoids rigidity, it is unlike most 'diet' plans out there. Make the 80–20 Plan the one you embrace moving forward so that you control your calorie intake in the long term. As you grow more accustomed to planning your meals using the 80–20 Plan, you will soon find it becomes a natural way of eating. You will naturally think as you eat, taking account of what you are putting into your body. Your fuel will mostly be made up of good wholesome healthy foods with the odd bit of 'junk' thrown in for good measure so you're not living life denying yourself the odd pleasure!

In using the plan, make sure you keep low-calorie snacks in the house and at work, such as low-cal dips with fruit or raw vegetables, as well as making sure you have water on tap. People often fall off the wagon and put the weight back on because they find traditional dieting too boring. With this in mind it's important to include some tasty healthy foods in your 80–20 Plan, such as tomatoes, strawberries, raspberries, blackberries, grapes, watermelon, sweet potatoes, roast potatoes cooked in low-calorie oil and some good lean meats, such as fish, chicken breast and turkey.

There are many other tasty foods, as you will note in my 80–20 Plan below. As you move forward with a slimmer body, build into your plan some daily motion. This doesn't mean you have to go to the gym for the rest of your life because let's face it, you may not have the time, but doing something that gets you moving a little really is important, even if it's just walking round the block before you go to bed, something I advocate as it also helps you sleep. Here's another example of an 80–20 Plan prepared for one of my clients. As you will see, you can mix and match the meal plans to suit you, week by week. This example will also help you understand further how to construct your own meal plans during the coming months.

The 6-week plan

6 WEEK PLAN	BREAKFAST	LUNCH	DINNER	SNACK ON...	A LITTLE OF WHAT YOU FANCY
Day 1: Monday	35g (1¼oz) porridge oats made with semi-skimmed milk. Serve with a drizzle of honey and grated apple.	50g (2oz) low-fat pâté served with two slices wholemeal toast and a large sliced tomato, plus a glass of orange juice.	Grill a portion of salmon and enjoy with a large serving of mixed salad leaves and eight new potatoes.	A crunchy apple or a nice cuppa with semi-skimmed milk.	Two plain biscuits.
Day 2: Tuesday	Two medium sized eggs (scrambled) on whole-meal toast, plus one apple.	A can of chunky vegetable soup with a wholemeal roll.	Stir-fry half a packet of stir-fry vegetables and add half a jar of sweet and sour sauce. Serve with an 80g (3¼oz) portion of cooked noodles.	A banana.	One toasted crumpet spread with 1 tsp low-fat spread.

6 WEEK PLAN	BREAKFAST	LUNCH	DINNER	SNACK ON...	A LITTLE OF WHAT YOU FANCY
Day 3: Wednesday	In a blender, whizz together a banana milkshake with 1 large ripe banana and 300ml (½ pint) semi-skimmed milk. Serve with a slice of wholemeal toast spread thinly with low-fat spread.	Grate 4 tbsp half-fat Cheddar and use to fill a medium-sized wholemeal roll; add a spoonful of low-fat crunchy coleslaw.	A portion of Skinny Chilli (see page 74) with a choice of two of your favourite vegetables.	A handful of grapes or a small skinny latte and two plain biscuits.	Baked or 'Lite' packet crisps to enjoy with your sandwich at lunchtime.
Day 4: Thursday	Spread a toasted wholemeal muffin with 1 tbsp low-fat cream cheese and top with a slice of smoked salmon, plus one apple or pear.	Grab a low-fat ready made chicken salad and fruit salad from your local store.	Grill two lean lamb chops and serve with a small baked potato and freshly cooked green beans.	2 tbsp low-fat cottage cheese on two crackers, plus one orange.	Two delicious scoops low-fat ice cream.
Day 5: Friday	25g (1oz) muesli with 2 tbsp raisins and semi-	Roast Beef Jacket: two slices lean roast beef with	Grilled chicken breast (skin removed) served with eight	Two small chocolate-chip	Enjoy your favourite tipple

6 WEEK PLAN	BREAKFAST	LUNCH	DINNER	SNACK ON...	A LITTLE OF WHAT YOU FANCY
	skimmed milk, plus a glass of juice.	one jacket potato, a handful of salad leaves and 2tbsp fat-free dressing; glass of juice.	new potatoes and lots of broccoli and carrots.	cookies or one crunchy apple.	– this may be a glass of wine, a beer or spirit with a slim-line mixer.
Day 6: Saturday	Low-fat Sausage Sandwich: Grill two low-fat sausages and serve between two slices of wholemeal bread with a sliced tomato.	A small can of tomato soup, served with two slices wholemeal toast to dip in! (skip the spread and use Marmite instead).	Curry Night Treat! Skip the starters and go for two poppadoms instead. Enjoy your favourite curry with plain boiled rice and a vegetable curry side order (no Bhaji or Naan!).	A banana or a handful of grapes.	
Day 7: Sunday	Two grilled tomatoes served on a thick slice of wholemeal or granary toast, with a rasher of grilled back bacon.	Tuck into a Lean Roast Dinner (see page 90).	Canned sardines on a thick slice of wholemeal toast with a few cherry tomatoes.	A nice cuppa with semi-skimmed milk and two plain biscuits or an orange.	A glass of your favourite tipple.

233

6 WEEK PLAN	BREAKFAST	LUNCH	DINNER	SNACK ON...	A LITTLE OF WHAT YOU FANCY
Day 8: Monday	25g (1oz) muesli with semi-skimmed milk and grapes, glass of juice and one banana.	Toss together a small can of tuna flakes (drained) with some diced cucumber and a handful of cherry tomatoes. Serve on salad leaves with 1 tbsp low-fat French dressing.	Jacket potato with a warmed small can of prepared ratatouille served with 15g (½oz) grated half-fat Cheddar and a small bowl of crunchy mixed salad.	A piece of fruit or a small handful of almonds.	
Day 9: Tuesday	McDonald's Double Bacon & Egg McMuffin or a scrambled egg on wholemeal toast with two rashers of grilled back bacon.	Fill a wholemeal roll with two slices lean ham and a large sliced tomato, plus one banana.	Light Macaroni Cheese (see page 73) with a handful of lean diced ham, served with two choices of vegetable.	A small skinny latte or a nice cuppa and a plain biscuit, plus one orange.	
Day 10: Wednesday	Two chocolate Weetabix with semi-skimmed milk and chunks of sliced banana.	Flake a mackerel fillet and serve with low-fat dressing over mixed salad leaves,	Two-egg ham and tomato omelette: use one slice of ham and one sliced	Shop-bought fruit smoothie or one apple.	Small piece chocolate cake.

6 WEEK PLAN	BREAKFAST	LUNCH	DINNER	SNACK ON...	A LITTLE OF WHAT YOU FANCY
		tomatoes and cucumber.	tomato. Serve with a large green salad.		
Day 11: Thursday	Dip chunky wedges of wholemeal toast soldiers (two slices) into two medium sized soft-boiled eggs.	Croque Monsieur (see page 91).	Grilled fresh tuna steak, eight new potatoes (boiled) and a huge bowl of mixed salad.	Carrot sticks and a small pot of low-fat dip; a banana.	
Day 12: Friday	Peanut butter on wholemeal toast, plus chunks of fruit (try pineapple and strawberries) with low-fat yoghurt.	A serving of Perfect Pea Soup (see page 76) with two wholemeal crackers or a slice of wholemeal bread.	Lean grilled beefsteak with Skinny Chips (see page 73). Serve with carrots and green beans.	A nice cuppa with semi-skimmed milk and two plain biscuits or a fun-size packet dried fruit.	A glass of your favourite tipple.

6 WEEK PLAN	BREAKFAST	LUNCH	DINNER	SNACK ON...	A LITTLE OF WHAT YOU FANCY
Day 13: Saturday	Poached egg on wholemeal toast and a glass of orange juice.	Wholemeal pitta filled with tuna and low-fat mayo mixed with diced cucumber and pepper.	Takeaway Treat: fish and chips from the local chippy! Choose a small portion and share the chips with a friend.	Two pieces of fruit.	
Day 14: Sunday	BLT – Two slices wholemeal bread filled with two rashers lean back bacon (grilled), lettuce, tomato and 2 tsp reduced-calorie mayonnaise; a piece of fruit.	Tuck into a Lean Roast Dinner (see page 90).	Three wholegrain crackers (for example, Ryvita), 25g (1oz) Brie and a baked apple. To bake the apple, preheat the oven to 200°C (400°F) Gas 6. Meanwhile, remove the core from a cooking apple and fill with raisins or sultanas. Add 1 tsp low-fat spread and bake for 20–25 minutes.	One banana.	A glass of your favourite tipple.

6 WEEK PLAN	BREAKFAST	LUNCH	DINNER	SNACK ON...	A LITTLE OF WHAT YOU FANCY
Day 15: Monday	25g (1oz) muesli with 2 tbsp raisins and semi-skimmed milk, plus a glass of juice.	Half a can of minestrone soup, slice of wholemeal toast with 3 tbsp grated half-fat Cheddar melted over the top.	6 tbsp cooked wholemeal pasta served with readymade tomato or vegetable sauce and a small can of flaked tuna or salmon (drained).	One apple.	Indulge yourself with a low-calorie hot chocolate and a plain biscuit.
Day 16: Tuesday	Indulge yourself with a low-calorie hot chocolate and a plain biscuit.	Jacket potato with 125g (4oz) cooked prawns mixed with 2 tbsp low-fat cocktail sauce.	Grilled pork chop (fat removed), served with mash (boil and mash one potato with 3 tbsp semi-skimmed milk), broccoli and carrots.	A small skinny latte or an apple.	
Day 17: Wednesday	Enjoy a large bowl of fruit salad (try apple, grapes and mango). Serve with a small pot of low-fat natural yoghurt.	Wholemeal pitta filled with sliced chicken and mixed salad.	A portion of Skinny Chilli (see page 74) with two choices of vegetable.	Two pieces of fruit.	

237

6 WEEK PLAN	BREAKFAST	LUNCH	DINNER	SNACK ON...	A LITTLE OF WHAT YOU FANCY
Day 18: Thursday	35g (1½oz) porridge oats or a ready measured sachet made with semi-skimmed milk, plus one apple.	Enjoy a Salade Niçoise (see page 96).	Lean grilled gammon steak with 4 tbsp mixed vegetables and a small portion of oven chips.	Fun-size packet dried raisins or apricots. Carrot sticks and a small pot of low-fat hummus.	
Day 19: Friday	McDonald's Egg McMuffin or poached egg on toast with a large regular black or white coffee.	A serving of Perfect Pea Soup (see page 76) with a granary roll.	Try our Homemade Turkey Burger in a bun (see page 78).	A handful of grapes or one apple.	A glass of your favourite tipple.
Day 20: Saturday	Try our skinny grilled English breakfast: Tuck into two slices of back bacon, mushrooms and tomatoes (spray with a little oil first). Serve with low-sugar baked beans.	Half an avocado filled with a small can of white crabmeat (drained). Serve with mixed salad leaves.	A portion of Skinny Chips (see page 73) served with a grilled lean beef steak and green beans.	One banana or a small pot of low-fat yoghurt.	Two scoops of sorbet.

6 WEEK PLAN	BREAKFAST	LUNCH	DINNER	SNACK ON...	A LITTLE OF WHAT YOU FANCY
Day 21: Sunday	Whizz up two scrambled eggs on a toasted crumpet. Serve with a glass of juice.	Tuck into a Lean Roast Dinner (see page 90).	Stir-fry a small packet of ready prepared vegetables and add 3 tbsp black bean sauce. Serve with 80g (3¼oz) cooked brown rice.	One orange or a small bunch of grapes.	Your favourite tipple.
Day 22: Monday	Low-fat Sausage Sandwich (see page 23).	Jacket potato with low-sugar baked beans and a glass of orange juice.	Enjoy a 'ready prepared' low-fat vegetable curry.	One banana.	One low-sugar fruit jelly.
Day 23: Tuesday	Enjoy a Lean Bacon Butty (see page 87).	Mixed Bean Salad: Drain and rinse a can of mixed beans. Transfer to a bowl and stir in 3 tbsp defrosted mixed vegetables. Crumble over 25g (1oz) feta cheese and serve with 1 tbsp low-fat dressing.	Serve a steaming bowl of freshly cooked tagliatelle with 125g (4oz) mixed seafood sautéed in a spray of oil and crushed garlic.	Two oatcakes or a nice cuppa and two plain biscuits.	

6 WEEK PLAN	BREAKFAST	LUNCH	DINNER	SNACK ON...	A LITTLE OF WHAT YOU FANCY
Day 24: Wednesday	Chocolate Weetabix with semi-skimmed milk and a handful of raspberries.	Wholemeal pasta salad made with cooked pasta, chopped peppers and cucumber, flaked canned salmon (drained) and 1 tbsp low-fat dressing.	Grilled pork chop (fat removed) with a large helping of ratatouille.	Two plain biscuits or an apple.	
Day 25: Thursday	Toasted bagel topped with 1 tbsp crunchy peanut butter and banana slices.	Two slices lean pork in a toasted wholemeal pitta with 1 tbsp low-cal coleslaw.	Grill a portion of salmon and enjoy with a large serving of mixed salad leaves and eight new potatoes.	One apple.	Indulge in a small bag of your favourite crisps.
Day 26: Friday	Dip chunky wedges of wholemeal toast soldiers (two slices) into two medium sized soft-boiled eggs.	Croque Monsieur (see page 91).	Make a tasty Lean Toad in the Hole (see page 75). Serve with freshly cooked carrots and peas.	A small pot of low-fat fruit yoghurt or one banana.	A glass of your favourite tipple.

6 WEEK PLAN	BREAKFAST	LUNCH	DINNER	SNACK ON...	A LITTLE OF WHAT YOU FANCY
Day 27: Saturday	5g (1oz) muesli with 2 tbsp chopped dried apricots, semi-skimmed milk and a glass of juice.	Enjoy a smoked salmon sandwich with shredded green lettuce between two slices of wholemeal bread.	Homemade Curry: Heat 1 tsp oil in a pan and fry 150g (5oz) sliced chicken breast (skin removed) and a selection of vegetables until golden. Add half a jar of low-fat korma curry sauce and cook for a further 15 minutes. Serve with 6 tbsp cooked brown rice.	A piece of fruit or a small handful of almonds.	Two delicious scoops low-fat ice cream.
Day 28: Sunday	Grilled tomatoes on one slice of wholemeal toast with a rasher of grilled back bacon on the side, plus a glass of orange juice.	Enjoy an egg mayo sandwich with shredded green lettuce between two slices of wholemeal bread.	A portion of Low-Cal Cottage Pie (see page 69) with two choices of vegetable.	Two pieces of fruit.	Enjoy a glass of your favourite tipple.

241

6 WEEK PLAN	BREAKFAST	LUNCH	DINNER	SNACK ON...	A LITTLE OF WHAT YOU FANCY
Day 29: Monday	Two toasted crumpets with low-sugar jam or marmalade and a nice cuppa made with semi-skimmed milk.	50g (2oz) low-fat pâté on a slice of wholemeal toast and one carrot, cut into sticks.	Make your favourite Lean Spaghetti Bolognese recipe using turkey mince (see page 88). Serve with 6 tbsp cooked wholemeal pasta and broccoli.	One banana or carrot sticks.	
Day 30: Tuesday	25g (1oz) muesli with 2 tbsp raisins and semi-skimmed milk, plus one banana and a glass of juice.	Pasta salad made with cooked wholemeal pasta, one slice of ham (cut into strips), chopped peppers and cucumber and 1 tbsp low-fat dressing – perfect for a lunchbox!	Grilled salmon fillet with roasted vegetables. To roast the vegetables, preheat the oven to 200°C (400°F) Gas 6. Meanwhile, deseed a pepper and cut into chunks, along with a courgette and a small onion. Spray with a little oil and roast for 20 minutes.	Two oatcakes or one apple.	One small piece of chocolate cake or chocolate bar (25g/1oz).

6 WEEK PLAN	BREAKFAST	LUNCH	DINNER	SNACK ON...	A LITTLE OF WHAT YOU FANCY
Day 31: Wednesday	Poached egg on a slice of wholemeal toast and a glass of orange juice.	Jacket potato with a small tub of cottage cheese and pineapple.	A portion of Low-Cal Cottage Pie (see page 69). Serve with two choices of vegetable.	One orange or a small bunch of grapes.	
Day 32: Thursday	35g (1½oz) porridge oats or a ready measured sachet made with semi-skimmed milk; one apple.	Wholemeal pitta filled with tuna and sweetcorn mixed with 1 tbsp low-fat mayo.	6 tbsp cooked wholemeal pasta served with readymade vegetable sauce.	A nice cuppa with a reduced-fat digestive or one apple.	
Day 33: Friday	Toasted wholemeal English muffin spread with 1 tbsp peanut butter, plus one apple.	Small can of minestrone soup with two wholemeal crackers.	Takeaway Treat! Enjoy a large takeout Thin & Crispy Vegetable & Ham Pizza.	One banana, one orange or two satsumas.	A large glass of your favourite tipple.
Day 34: Saturday	A small bowl of Bran Flakes or 2 Weetabix served with a handful of	In a bowl, toss together a small can of salmon (drained and flaked) with	Grilled chicken breast (skin removed), served with eight new potatoes and	Two oatcakes with 2 tbsp cottage cheese or carrot sticks.	Low-fat chocolate mousse for a dinner-time dessert.

6 WEEK PLAN	BREAKFAST	LUNCH	DINNER	SNACK ON...	A LITTLE OF WHAT YOU FANCY
	strawberries and semi-skimmed milk.	half a diced pepper and a handful of sliced cherry tomatoes. Serve on salad leaves.	lots of broccoli and carrots.		
Day 35: Sunday	Lean Bacon Butty (see page 87).	Tuck into a Lean Roast Dinner (see page 90).	Two-egg omelette with half-fat Cheddar and a large mixed salad. Stew some cooking apples and serve with a small pot of yoghurt for dessert.	Fun-size pack of dried fruit or three breadsticks.	Enjoy a glass of your favourite tipple.
Day 36: Monday	Poached egg on wholemeal toast served with grilled tomatoes and a glass of juice.	Mackerel Pâté (see page 71) on a slice of wholemeal toast. Ready prepared fruit salad or fruit yoghurt.	Serve a steaming bowl of freshly cooked tagliatelle with 125g (4oz) mixed seafood sautéed with a handful of spinach in a spray of oil and crushed garlic.	A nice cuppa made with semi-skimmed milk and a plain biscuit or one apple.	

6 WEEK PLAN	BREAKFAST	LUNCH	DINNER	SNACK ON...	A LITTLE OF WHAT YOU FANCY
Day 37: Tuesday	Tuck into a bowl of chopped apple and pineapple served with a dollop of Greek yoghurt (0 per cent fat).	Grab a ready prepared chicken salad and a tub of fruit salad.	Two grilled lean lamb chops served with a can of warmed ratatouille.	One banana.	A bar of milk chocolate (25g/1oz).
Day 38: Wednesday	Two scrambled eggs on a slice of wholemeal toast, plus a glass of orange juice.	Hummus Wrap: Spread a flour tortilla with 3 tbsp low-fat hummus. Top with shredded lettuce and slices of cucumber and tomato. Tuck in the ends, roll up and enjoy!	6 tbsp cooked wholemeal pasta served with readymade tomato sauce with 3 tbsp mixed vegetables.	Two oatcakes or one piece of fruit.	
Day 39: Thursday	Chocolate Weetabix with semi-skimmed milk and a handful of raspberries.	Two slices lean pork in a toasted wholemeal pitta with 1 tbsp low-cal coleslaw.	Grilled salmon fillet, served with 80g (3¼oz) cooked brown rice with 2 tbsp pesto stirred through. Serve with green beans or spinach.	Fun-size packet of dried fruit or carrot sticks.	

6 WEEK PLAN	BREAKFAST	LUNCH	DINNER	SNACK ON...	A LITTLE OF WHAT YOU FANCY
Day 40: Friday	McDonald's Big Breakfast and one apple.	Jacket potato with a warmed can of ratatouille and 15g (½oz) grated half-fat Cheddar.	A portion of Lean Toad in the Hole (see page 75), served with freshly cooked carrots and green beans.	One orange.	Two Jaffa Cakes or indulge in a small bag of your favourite crisps with lunch, or your favourite tipple.
Day 41: Saturday	Low-Fat Sausage Sandwich (see page 231).	Can of lentil soup and a wholemeal bread roll.	A portion of Skinny Chilli (see page 74) with two choices of vegetable.	Small bunch grapes or carrot sticks.	
Day 42: Sunday	Low-sugar baked beans on wholemeal toast	A portion of Low-Cal Cottage Pie (see page 69), served with two choices of vegetable.	Sardines on a thick slice of wholemeal toast with cucumber slices.	Two pieces of fruit.	A glass of your favourite tipple.

TAKE THE IMMEDIATE STEPS

So, having read almost to the end of this book you may be wondering how to get started. Perhaps you're feeling a little lost in terms of what needs to be done to start your own weight-loss program and so in this, the final chapter, I'd like to offer you an example of what to do in your first week. You may use this as a working example and edit to suit you. It will help get you focused and into the zone to move forward for the long haul. Remember, this is not just another faddy diet – it's about helping you to lose the weight and keep it off for good! As you move forward right now, look on it as a complete change in lifestyle designed to help you become the person you want to be, and also deserve to be. During your first week, together we will develop a plan to put things in place and this will help you to develop a positive attitude and a belief in yourself, as well as a long-term capability to win the war on fat, so read on!

SUNDAY

- Okay, write down all the excuses you have been
  making over the years for not losing weight. Once
  you have listed them, look closely at each one.
  Admit to yourself that it is these excuses that have
  kept you fat and at last you are letting go of them
  for good. Finally, tear them up and put them in the
  bin.

- Develop a couple of positive affirmations to say to
  yourself daily that will remind you that you are
  becoming more in control of food and losing
  weight successfully (see page 13). If it helps, write
  them down in big block capitals on bright card and
  place around the house where you will see them
  daily.

- Design your 80–20 meal plans for the forthcoming
  week (see page 67) and prepare a shopping list to
  get everything you need to make them from the
  supermarket. Remember to include the odd treat
  because denial, as you may well know, is totally
  doomed! You are now entering a lifestyle change as
  opposed to a crash diet that would probably result
  in you putting all the weight back on, so the 80–20
  Plan will make it real for you.

MONDAY

- Visit the supermarket and purchase all you need
  to make your meal plans for the week. If you
  work full time, you might ask a friend or family
  member to do this for you or alternatively, shop
  online.

- Decide what exercise you will be doing on a daily

basis to help get your body moving, but as well as this, start thinking about a new exercise that you would like to do for leisure (see page 183).

- Practice relaxation and then visualise yourself slimmer, trimmer and healthier. Imagine this image embedded deep into your mind (see page 158). If you find this difficult, consider getting support from a certified clinical hypnotherapist (make sure you find someone who is reputable). Implement the first day of the 80–20 plan and consciously eat more slowly, taking occasional sips of water.

TUESDAY

- Today, think about those friends who are the drains in your life, the ones who sap your energy and prefer to talk about themselves constantly rather than asking about you, too. Then do the reverse by thinking about the radiators in your life, the people who give you time, never pull you down and have a general optimism about your weight loss. Think about how you can ignore the drains and spend more time with the radiators. For example, you may stop taking the calls from the drains or begin telling them that you are too busy to meet up. *Never* feel guilty!

- Observe the activities of fat people: notice what bad habits they have when it comes to food control and exercise. Deliberately watch them eating large portions and eating quickly. Notice how they struggle to move or sit comfortably in a seat and how simply walking soon causes breathlessness in them. Remember, it isn't the *person* you are judging, but the results of fat. Allow these observations to encourage you away from a life of fat.

- Today you may also want to pay special attention to portion control using the techniques outlined in the book (*see also* pages 84).
- Go walking (see page 186) and when you get home, enjoy a healthy meal from the plans you have developed.
- End the day by practicing some positive visualisation in which you see the end result – again, you looking slimmer and gorgeous! Afterwards, affirm you are in control of food and that you enjoy reducing your weight successfully (*see also* page 164).

WEDNESDAY

- If you notice yourself eating because of stress then identify from this book what will work best to help you alleviate it (see page 123). Identify what will help to control your emotional eating habit and take action!
- Tell a few good friends (the ones who are radiators) about your new way of eating but do not lend them this book! I want you to keep it right by your side as a constant source of support.
- If the family are becoming interested in what you are up to (and also need to lose weight), agree a family mission with them and then explain how the 80–20 plan works. Sit down together to agree all the actions you will take to successfully lose

weight together. Pin a list of these actions on the wall so that everyone sees them every day.

- Implement Day 4 of your 80–20 plan and once you have finished, take half an hour to let your meal go down before taking a walk. As you walk, reflect on how well you are doing and how as each day passes, you are moving away from a life of fat.

THURSDAY

- Get up early today and go for a 45-minute walk before work. When you get in, take a shower and think about how good it feels to be losing weight. Enjoy breakfast before leaving for work, or taking the kids to school.

- At work today remind yourself that weight loss is exciting! Deliberately notice or think about how most people will tell you that it's a real struggle. Now remind yourself that because you take responsibility, weight loss is exciting and will continue to be even more so as the days continue.

- Using your 80–20 plan notice how you can eat the odd bit of 'junk' but still have control over it.

- Take a longer walk after work before preparing your evening meal. Having decided on what exercise you would like to do for leisure, surf the Web because tomorrow you are going to arrange it or even get started. Alternatively, agree with the family that this weekend you will do something together that involves moving the body.

FRIDAY

- Think through an outfit that you would love to wear in a much smaller size. Imagine yourself in it and all the compliments you will receive.
- Dig out an old 'fat' photograph of yourself and keep this somewhere you can find it easily. Use this as a motivator, pushing you away from living the fat life again. Remind yourself that the past is the past.
- If possible, today take up your new exercise for pleasure regime or make arrangements for this. Maybe you have decided to play badminton or to go out and buy a table tennis kit for the whole family.
- Enjoy your evening meal with friends or family. Let them begin to understand how it works. If anyone tells you that it's hard to lose weight, adopt a cynical attitude and tell yourself that they will simply stay fat with that attitude!

SATURDAY

- Now it's time for you to go out today and buy your new outfit that's a size or two, or even three smaller (*see also* page 12). When you get home, hang it somewhere you will see it daily, ideally on the wardrobe so you notice it as soon as you get out of bed. Go on, treat yourself!
- Do some exercise with the family. Go for a good long walk and maybe finish with a picnic in the park (*see also* page 204).
- As it's the weekend, enjoy a nice 80–20 plan meal to include a couple of glasses of your favourite tipple. Reflect on the week and congratulate

yourself on doing well. You have achieved so much in the first week and now it's time to move forward for the rest of your life!

EVER THOUGHT ABOUT A CAREER AS A WEIGHT-LOSS COACH?

As you progress and the weight drops off you may find that your own journey inspires you to train as a weight-loss coach. The UK is now the fattest country in Europe and millions of people are seeking support. There is nothing more inspiring than being coached to lose weight by someone who has actually been fat themselves because they will understand the struggles and the negative feelings being overweight carries. Naturally, you will have bags of empathy and understand what is needed to lose weight effectively. If you want to train to become a weight-loss coach, it's important to find a reputable training provider.

Having been fat and having lost the weight – as well as developing the ability to control my weight and keep it off – led me to do just this and I now run a certificate in weight-loss coaching. There's nothing better than seeing people gain confidence and become more at peace with themselves as they learn to control their weight. If you want to continue the journey and are interested in training to become a weight-loss coach, visit thestevemillerplan.com for further details.

A FINAL WORD

So, there you have it. My secrets are revealed and it really is about having the right positive attitude, learning to behave as someone who is in control of their weight and finally, acquiring the capabilities of a successful slimmer. As you move forward into the future, I want you to take this book with you. If you have days when it becomes a struggle to eat wisely and exercise well, pick up the book and just read a chapter of it to help you overcome this temporary loss of focus. Remember, you do deserve it and it's all very possible. And now it's time for you to get excited about what will be. Remember, the best way to get a result is to take action, so start right now!